CONTENTS

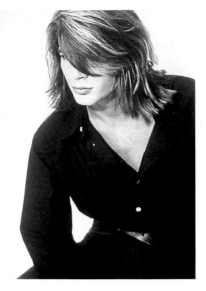

Charles Worthington

Foreword vi

Introduction vii

Acknowledgements viii

1 Style artistry 1
Introduction 1
How is an image created? 1
Creative style design 2
Analysing the essential style components 2

2 The total image 9
Introduction 9
Consultation 9
Assessing the total image 9

3 Professional consultation 18
Introduction 18
The purpose of consultation 18
The consultation process 19
After the consultation 25
Hair and skin tests 26
Hair and scalp diseases, conditions and defects 29

4 Creative cutting 37
Introduction 37
Graduated bob 38
Short contemporary graduation 42
Transient short layers 46
Short graduation 50
Square layers 54
Forward graduation 58
Cutting and styling 62
Cutting baselines 62
Cutting tools 63
Razor cut 65
Shaping and texturising 66
Accuracy and checks 67

5   Creative perming 71
Introduction 71
Twist and roll using hair formers 72
The background to perming 74
Perming techniques 78

6   Creative colouring 89
Introduction 89
Block highlights 90
Layered colour 92
Colour flashes 94
Asymmetric shimmer 96
Surface slices 98
Block colouring 100
Facial framing 102
Colouring principles 104
Hair colourants 106
Bleaching and lightening 110
Colour variations 113
Recolouring 115
Toning 116
Decolouring 118

7   Creative styling and dressing 119
Introduction 119
High knot 120
Low knot 122
Pleat 124
Plaiting 126
Weaving 128
Added hair – postiche 129
Attaching a hairpiece 130
Hair extensions 132
Ornamentation and hair accessories 139
Fashion setting techniques 140

8   African-Caribbean hair techniques 143
Introduction 143
Consultation 143
Styling hair using heated equipment 144
Routine and corrective hair relaxing services 146

9   Working as a team 151
Introduction 151
Getting organised 151
Effective communication 153
Working as a team 155
Personal development 156
The role of the supervisor 160
Disciplinary action 164

10 Finance and resources 168
Introduction 168
Human resources 168
Time resources 168
Physical resources 169
Financial resources 173
Productivity 180

11 Training 182
Introduction 182
The provision of training 182
Identifying training needs 184
Planning training 185
Delivering training 187
Supporting learners 189
Self-development 190

12 Assessment 192
Introduction 192
Standards of competence 192
Assessing trainees 195
Providing feedback 197

13 Salon promotion 199
Introduction 199
Promoting the business 199
Demonstrating services 202
Advertising 204
Photography 205

14 Health, safety and security 211
Introduction 211
Personal health and hygiene 212
General salon hygiene 215
Preventing infection 217
Working safely in the salon 217
Dealing with accidents 219
Fire 222
Maintaining salon security 224
Health and safety legislation 225
Writing a health and safety policy 229

Appendix 1 Portfolio guidance 230

Appendix 2 Accreditation of prior learning 232

Appendix 3 Useful addresses 233

Glossary 235

Index 239

A favourite saying of mine is best is not enough . . . only excellence will do!

Each and every day our organisation strives to improve upon our achievements of the previous day. We do this by focusing on the value we put upon learning, commitment and working together. With this, we can provide excellent customer service.

I believe one of the greatest things a person can do is to expand their knowledge and gain new skills. Yet these by themselves are worthless unless you have a goal in life. For some, Level 3 is that goal. For others, Level 3 is only the route to higher achievements. Be it goal or route, achieving this standard is immensely profitable.

Make learning part of your life. Say yes to knowledge. And remember, best is not enough . . . only excellence will do!

Alan Goldsbro
Chief Executive
Hairdressing Training Board

Lewis Dyer at Nicky Clarke

INTRODUCTION

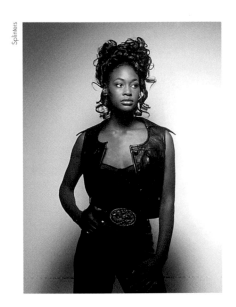

Splinters

This second edition of *Professional Hairdressing* has been completely rewritten and updated. It covers all the essential information for anyone preparing to undertake NVQ Level 3. It also provides an ideal companion for others who simply wish to improve on their own skills in the world of professional hairdressing.

NEW IDEAS

You will find that this book is set out in a different way to other books. We have arranged the essential aspects of planning and preparation of hairdressing in a logical and simplified format – as building blocks of information.

It's as easy as ABC. The system introduced in this book creates a pattern of thinking which ensures that all the essential aspects of communication and practical skills are comprehensively covered.

HOW TO USE THIS BOOK

This book has a modular format, with each chapter covering a specific area. Some chapters are artistic and creative, others practical and methodical. The remainder provide essential information for business development.

You can use this book with its free form in any order you like. We hope you enjoy using it and that it will prove to be an invaluable salon aid.

Note about pronouns

Using 'he or she' and 'him or her' throughout the text would become cumbersome in a book such as this. For simplicity and ease of reading, therefore, we have used simply 'she' and 'her' throughout.

Lesley Kimber

Martin Green

Leo Palladino

ACKNOWLEDGEMENTS

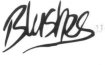
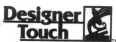
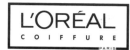
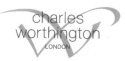
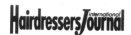
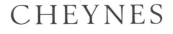
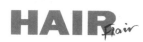

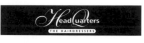
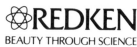
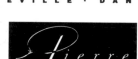
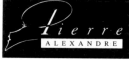
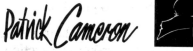
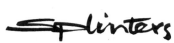

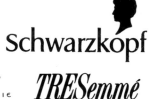

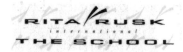

The authors and publishers would like to thank the following for providing pictures for the book: Alastair Hughes, Andrew Collinge, Best of British, BLM Health, Blushes, Charles Worthington, Charlie Taylor, Cheynes Training, Claire Fawlk, Clynol Hair, Depilex/RVB, Dome Cosmetics, Dr Andrew L Wright (Consultant Dermatologist, Bradford Royal Infirmary), Dr M H Beck (Consultant Dermatologist, Salford Royal Hospital NHS Trust), Ellisons, Fire Protection Service, Goldwell Hair Cosmetics Ltd, Great Lengths, Hair Flair, Hairdressers Journal International, Hairdressing Training Board, Headquarters, Ian Flanders, ICI, Joseph Roberts, Karen Turner, Lewis Dyer, L'Oréal Coiffure, Luster Products Inc. (Designer Touch), Mahogany, Neville Daniel, Nicky Clarke, Patrick Cameron, Pierre Alexandre, Redken, Regis, Rita Rusk, S Lewis, SAKS, Sam Cairney, Schwarzkopf, Smith & Nephew, Steve Whitfield of Freeze Frame Photography, Splinters Group, Terence Renati, The Controller of Her Majesty's Stationery Office for Crown Copyright Material, TRESemmé, Trevor Sorbie, Vidal Sassoon, Wella Great Britain, Zoe Mitchell.

Special thanks to Michelle Blake from The House of Colour, Gloucester, for her contribution on 'The Total Image'.

Every effort has been made to trace all the copyright holders, but if any have been inadvertently overlooked the publishers will be pleased to make the necessary arrangements at the first opportunity.

CHAPTER 1

Style artistry

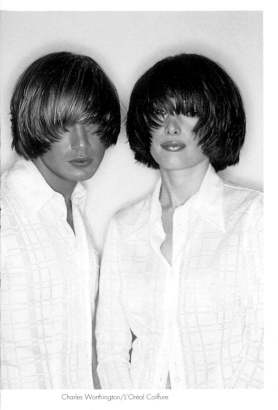

Charles Worthington/L'Oréal Coiffure

INTRODUCTION

'Style artistry' is a term associated with style, interpretation and design. It involves a variety of specialist skills:

- appreciation of shape, dimension, image, colour and textures
- understanding balance, imbalance, suitability and application
- expressing creativity by designing, moulding, shaping and forming the hair
- explaining visual interpretations to clients during consultation
- analysing what can be seen and touched
- manipulating and manoeuvring the hair into position.

Hair styling can be artistic, practical and scientific. A hairdresser who can bring together the skills of artistic perception, practical ability and sound knowledge will always be in demand by clients.

This chapter sets out to capture these essential components, helping you to build a picture from a jigsaw puzzle. Bit by bit, piece by piece, you will discover the building blocks of style artistry: a pattern of thinking.

HOW IS AN IMAGE CREATED?

'Image' is understood by different people in different ways. If we look the word up in a reference book, its meaning is given as 'representation, likeness, semblance, form, appearance, configuration and structure'. In general terms, an image is examined by our senses:

- sight
- hearing
- touch
- taste
- smell.

These senses enable us to form an overall impression.

Let's take a look at one particular image: the salon in which you work. What sort of image does it portray to the public? What do your clients 'sense'?

- *What do they see?* Is the salon in a basement or upstairs? Is it on the main high street or in a housing estate? What colour schemes have been used inside? Is this carried through in printed information, for instance cards, price lists and service information?

- *What do they hear?* How are they spoken to on the telephone? How are they greeted when they enter the salon? How are they received, directed and consulted afterwards? What background noise can they hear?
- *What do they feel?* Can they feel the quality of fresh towels and gowns? Can they feel the level of professional contact in the ways that services and treatments are carried out?
- *What can they smell?* What is the salon atmosphere like? What do the products used smell like? Do the staff smell clean and hygienic?
- *What can they taste?* Are they provided with any drink or food while they are in the salon?

The client will judge the levels of quality and professionalism within these individual aspects and form an overall impression. This book does not set out to define a total image for salons, but it should help you in creating total image concepts for your clients.

CREATIVE STYLE DESIGN

Creative style design is a process of logical analysis which sets out to achieve a 'personalised' overall appearance or image. This is rather like following a recipe. We use, mix, add and blend various essential ingredients, which *together* combine to take on a new form that is completely different from what we started with. If the recipe is followed carefully, the result can be guaranteed. If it is not, a disaster may occur.

A creative stylist can imagine the final effect and then work out the components needed to create that particular look. This increased level of expertise is what separates the creative and artistic stylist, who may be a specialist in certain hairdressing fields, from the average 'all-round' technician.

Salons do not need to employ specialists, and in many cases larger salon groups prefer to employ staff with all-round abilities. However, in progressive salons, where style directors are employed, we might expect them to pass their skills to others through training and developmental activities.

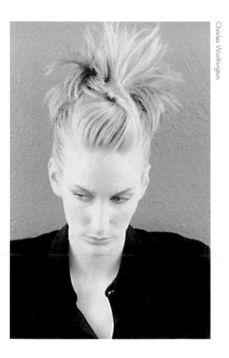

Charles Worthington

ANALYSING THE ESSENTIAL STYLE COMPONENTS

If you look at the style components in isolation, as building blocks, you will be able to approach the task of style artistry in a logical and systematic way.

Shape and form

Lines and angles

Adopted techniques

Apparent texture

Movement and direction

Dimensions, distribution and abundance

Colour depth and tone

Condition

Hair type

Method of operation

Specialised techniques

Moulding and shaping

Product application

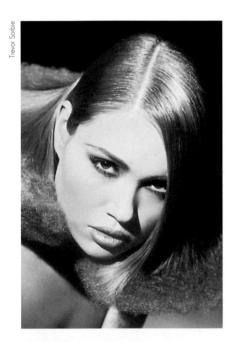

Trevor Sorbie

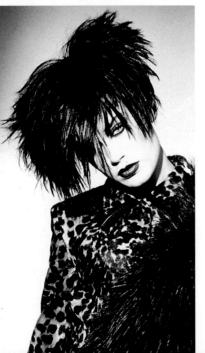

Roz Main at Rita Rusk

Shape and form

☐ Does the client have a photograph of the image she wants? How will this look in three dimensions?
☐ Will the overall effect be 'right' for the client's type of hair and features?

The overall effect is created by the structure of the underlying parts of the hair. This image is carefully composed of shape, form, direction and dimension.

As hairdressers, you must mentally interpret what you see. Often clients have specific styles in mind and may show you pictures to describe what they want. You must imagine a three-dimensional effect from a two-dimensional illustration. Getting this right, and relaying the information back to the client in a way that is easy to understand, is half the battle. This is an essential part of style composition and professional consultation.

Use your skills to fill in the missing information relating to contour, length, distribution of weight and proportions which will ultimately affect style suitability. Certain styles may be 'right' in that they enhance or accentuate the client's features. Others may be 'wrong' in that unsuitable effects spoil and undermine professional hairdressing disciplines.

Having analysed these overall impressions, you can dissect the style further into its component parts.

Lines and angles

☐ How does the line, the direction in which the hair is positioned, flow?

The perimeter of the hairstyle is formed by the outside line of the hair. The distance of this line from the scalp forms the depth of the shape. The lines and angles of the hair inside the perimeter affect the finished shape of the style. The hair outline forms semicircles which may be seen from the front, sides and back. The lines within this may be vertical, horizontal or crossing diagonally. These features help to create the visual effect.

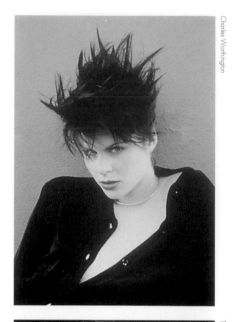

Charles Worthington

Adopted Techniques

How will you achieve the finished hairstyle?
How will this affect the style you create?

Hair can be styled and finished with a variety of techniques. Each has its own specific principles, allowing hair to be crafted and positioned in different ways.

You can create a range of different effects by using any one or a combination of blow drying, scrunch drying, finger or hand drying, stretching or straightening, backbrushing, backcombing, teasing, wet or dry setting, and tonging. These techniques can be used to lift, smooth, bend or flatten hair. Individually or collectively, they contribute to the inner and outer style structure and directions in which the hair moves.

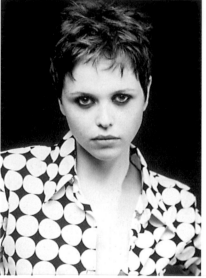

Trevor Sorbie

Apparent texture

☐ What is the texture of the individual hairs? How do they look and feel?
☐ What is the texture of the hair as a whole? How does it look and feel?
☐ How will this affect the finished look?

Texture is the term given to the way an object feels: rough or smooth; fine or coarse. In hairdressing, we can see the visual textural effects and we can also feel the textural aspects.

At NVQ Level 2 you were required to analyse individual hair textures, but at the higher levels of understanding you need to look holistically at the impact that texture has within and on the whole hairstyle.

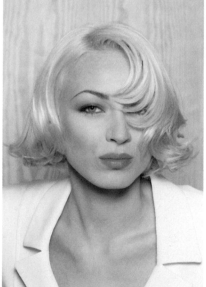

SAKS

Movement and direction

☐ What direction will the cut have?
☐ Will it be made up of flowing or broken lines of movement?

The direction that the hairs take, individually and collectively, affects the overall style. The position and line of the hair gives direction to the style. The variation of this line produces direction within the style. The more varied the line direction, the more

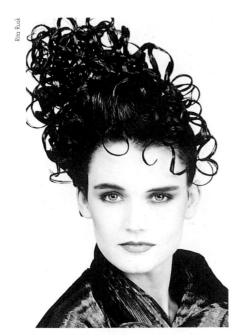

Rita Rusk

movement will be seen, showing as texture, wave or curl.

A fluid or flowing line gives a softer effect, whereas broken lines of movement create a harder visual impact. The more breaks within the style continuity, the greater the contrasts produced.

Dimensions, distribution and abundance

- What are the hair dimensions: is it wide, high, or does it have depth?
- What is the natural distribution and abundance of the hair?

The dimensions of a style are formed by the height at which the hair is positioned, the width of the bulk of the hair, and the depth of the style. The length of the hair gives the visual effects of perimeter line and internal style structure.

The hair's natural abundance and distribution pattern are also important. Height can make round faces look longer; width can broaden a thin face; hair can be angled away from or towards extreme features to make them look bigger or smaller. However, it is essential to remember that there is a limit to what can be done.

The number of actively growing hairs on a client's head is a basic element in deciding on style and shape, as well as taking into consideration texture, length, hair type and patterns of growth. You should consider hair whorls or distinctive growth patterns before attempting to cut or style. This can reduce the chance of error in style planning. There may be places where the hair grows abundantly, or not at all. Alternatively, you may see whole heads of sparse or thickly growing hair. All these eventualities need careful consideration.

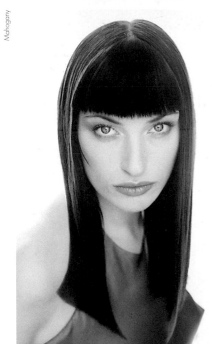

Mahogany

Colour depth and tone

- How light and dark is the hair? How light or dark could you make it?
- Remember that hair colour, tone and hue are as important to shape as lines and angles are to cutting.

Lightness and darkness, shade and shadow, harmonious and discordant colour, tints and hues create a varied range of effects which highlight or encompass the hair shape.

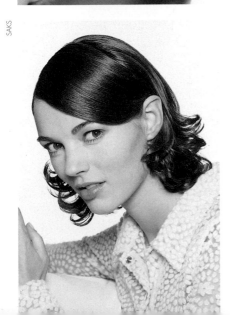

SAKS

Condition

- What condition is the hair in?
- Does it need treatment before you start styling?

The condition of the hair – its state of health – affects most of the other style components. It directly affects all aspects of style choice, and also the durability and manageability of the hairstyle to be created.

Poor hair health should be discussed with the client and stabilised or adjusted before any other procedures are carried out.

Hair type

- What hair type are you dealing with?
- If it is African-Caribbean or very dark hair, it will require careful chemical treatment.

Hair types fall into three main categories: Caucasian, Mongoloid and African-Caribbean.

Caucasian (European) hair is usually loosely waved or straight, and can range in colour from light to dark brown. It has a medium, soft texture.

Mongoloid (Asian) hair tends to be straight and lank. Its colour ranges from darkest black to mid-brown. The texture is predominantly coarse, and so chemical treatments are usually more complex on this type of hair.

African-Caribbean hair is usually tightly kinked or curly. Again, darker hair colouring is more predominant, requiring careful chemical treatment.

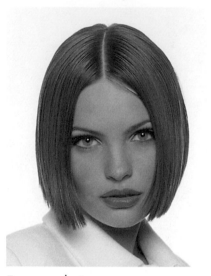

European hair

Method of operation

- Follow an orderly sequence of operation in all hairdressing procedures.
- Haphazard working techniques will result in mistakes and failures.
- Make sure you feel comfortable while you work.
- Follow the manufacturer's advice where possible.

Methods of creating different style effects vary, and there is usually more than one route to achieving the required effect. If you apply your chosen method systematically, it can be repeated if and when it is required again.

You will not be successful if you attempt to achieve style and shape without prior thought and consideration. This kind of haphazard and confused work will usually result in failure. Different and new ways of application can be tried when experimenting on models.

You should ensure that you are comfortable while you work: minimise stress and strain, keep your hand positions relaxed, and make sure your tools are comfortable to hold. Select those that enable you to achieve the specific effect you require.

Methods of application of chemical products are recommended by the manufacturers and these must be followed. They will have

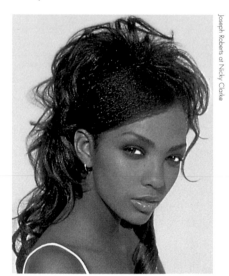

African-Caribbean hair

Roz Main at Rita Rusk

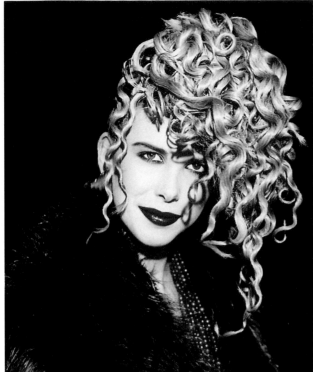

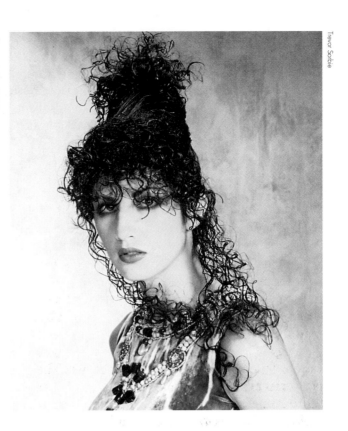

Trevor Sorbie

tried and tested the best methods before the products are released for sale and public use.

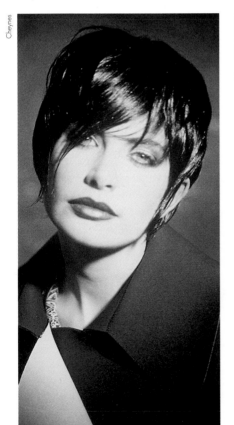

Cheynes

Specialised techniques

☐ Decide which effects you want to create before you start.
☐ Remember, there are mechanical aids to hair styling as well as chemical, permanent ones.

Hair moulding, shaping, finger waving, curling, plaiting, pleating, twisting and weaving can all be used to create special styling effects.

Rollers, velcro-rollers, flexible foam-covered rollers, Lockwell formers, pins and clips are the tools of hair shaping, and you must decide which effects are required before you apply these tools. These are the mechanical aids to hair styling, and are additional to the chemical tools and techniques now available.

Moulding and shaping

☐ Shaping and forming is cutting and moulding.
☐ Hair symmetry should be pleasing and harmonious.

Some types of hair can now be styled in ways which were previously impossible. Unruly hair can now be tamed, and difficult hair can achieve realistic shapes.

STYLE ARTISTRY   **7**

To shape and form hair is to cut and mould – to create. This involves the distribution of portions of hair into fitting outlines and positions. 'Proportioning' the hair means arranging and fitting it to the underlying head and face foundation. The outline shape or silhouette can be viewed from different directions and the balanced symmetry of the hair shape should generally be pleasing and harmonious.

Product application

- Choose which hair products you intend to use.
- Remember that there are many different products which can help to volumise hair.
- Read the manufacturer's instructions carefully.

Special and careful consideration needs to be given to hair products. Their contribution to styling makes them an additional hair-crafting tool.

As well as the vast range of shampoos and washes, internal and external conditioners, dressings and moisturisers available, you can now create texture, volume and movement by using a variety of gels, sculpting creams, moulding mousses, fixing waves, hair thickeners and other hair controllers.

To gain the maximum benefit from these products, it is vital to know how they should be used and applied. Always study the manufacturer's instructions.

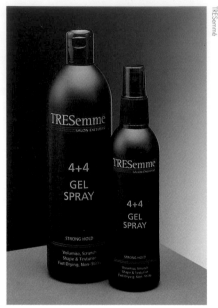

Hair products

ASSIGNMENT

Forthcoming trends for hairstyles appear in both trade and consumer publications. Make a visit to your high street newsagent and find out what will be the next trends within hairdressing fashions.

In your portfolio, make notes with illustrations of the future looks. Make sure that you give a full explanation in relation to effects, cuts, lengths, colour, perms and texture.

QUESTIONS

After you have completed the assignment, answer these questions in your portfolio.

1 What magazines did you use within your study?
2 In what ways do future fashions differ from current hairdressing looks?
3 Name the hairdressers or hairdressing

companies that were involved in predicting future trends within those publications.
4 In what other ways do these hairdressers promote hair styling to:
  a) the hairdressing industry?
  b) the public?

CHAPTER 2

The total image

Lewis Dyer at Nicky Clarke

INTRODUCTION

Total image is the general impression we receive of an individual person. It is made up of shape, form, dimension and colour. It is influenced by personality, nature, attitude and bearing. More specifically, total image is hair shape and style, fabric, fashion, physique, clothes and accessories.

All these elements reflect the visual presentation of the individual person. When you first meet a client, you react according to what you see, hear or interpret. Both the client and the stylist make an impression on each other and respond to each other accordingly.

CONSULTATION

The aim of consultation is to arrive at a suitable hairstyle or hair colour which is pleasing to the client. This should be done in a way that gives the client confidence in the salon and in you. The process should be inspiring.

It is necessary to study the 'complete picture' when you first meet the client. This is to make sure that you have enough information to advise her properly. Your aim is not to alter what the client wears or her self-image, but to harmonise with these to achieve satisfaction.

Consider all the aspects of the client's existing image and ask yourself what your impression is. Is there anything that doesn't work? Is the client happy with the existing style? She may point to areas which you feel are wrong, and you must explain your perspective with understanding.

ASSESSING THE TOTAL IMAGE

The total look should be individual to each client. It is designed as we cut and shape the hair. We add volume or colour to enhance the style, and blow dry or dress the hair. We consider hair type, natural colour and face shape, storing and applying all this information to build the total image. If we then add colour knowledge and image knowledge, we are closer to a look which should please the client. We should consult the client to find out about her personal image, lifestyle and personality, as well as the amount of time she can give to her hair. If we assess this carefully, we will arrive at a successful result every time.

Hairdressers are part of a world of images. We are asked for guidance and understanding of hairstyle, colour fashion and all that relates to the achievement of the total image.

Total image is made up of many building blocks. Together these create a whole impression. We will look at them separately so we can study their contribution more carefully.

Facial expression

Hair

Face and head shape

Eyes

Ears, nose and mouth

Make-up

Neck and shoulders

Hands

Body shape

Lifestyle and personality

Colour

Clothes and accessories

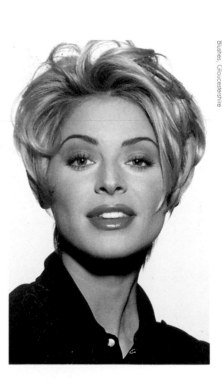

Blushes, Gloucestershire

Facial expression

- Always make eye contact with your client.
- Note your client's expression and react to it appropriately.

Facial expression is an important part of communication. Even if your client looks disgruntled or is scowling, use a friendly, pleasant expression to encourage her to relax. Facial expression is part of the total image, because it reflects the client's mood or how she is feeling. You need to pick up on these expressions and react to them appropriately. In this way you will understand the client's wants and needs more easily.

Hair

- Look at what kind of hair your client has.
- If the hair is fine, remember that most clients want volume which will last, which means using volumising cutting techniques.
- Consider proportioning the hair weight.
- Is your client trying to project a certain image: trendy, traditional?

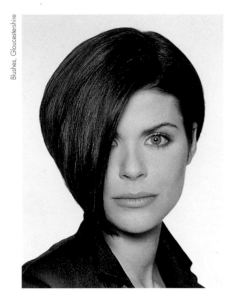

Face shapes
(a) Soft

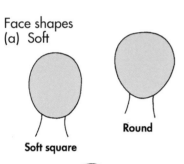

Soft square

Round

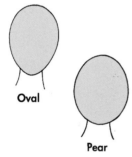

Oval

Pear

(b) Straight or cornered

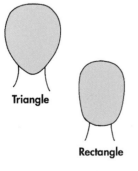

Triangle

Rectangle

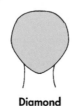

Diamond

After noting the client's facial expressions, you should move on to look at her hair. Length, quantity, quality and texture of the hair all contribute to the total image.

Fine hair often lacks body; most clients want fullness and volume which will last. Cutting methods to achieve this include volumising techniques, where body can be created by using longer layers levelled in line with the client's baselines and face shape.

You should also consider proportioning the hair weight. By setting hair and using light perms, you can create bulk and volume which give foundation to shape and style.

Hair fashion is constantly changing, and the client who wears a hairstyle which is of the moment wants to give the impression of being in touch with trends. Sometimes clients want up-to-the-minute hairstyles to keep a youthful image or to make themselves feel confident.

People often choose a particular image that complements their career and lifestyle. Television presenters, solicitors and newscasters may go for fashionable but traditional looks. Models will display the current themes. Those in artistic careers may choose very avant-garde styles. Some of these fashions may be durable, but many are fleeting.

Face and head shape

What shape is your client's face? Is it rounded or angular?
How large or small is the head?
What is the profile of the head like?

The basic, natural shape of the head, face and features are what form the underlying structure in styling. The proportions of the hair mass and distribution in relation to the face and head are vital in choosing a style. The outer hair shape should fit the face shape to achieve a suitable hair arrangement.

The contours of the head are its focal points. Those on the side of the head are formed by the parietal and temporal bones. Those on the back of the head and the nape are formed by the occipital bones, which can be *concave* or *convex*: curving inwards or outwards. The frontal bone forms the forehead shape. It is the beginning of the profile, which follows along the nose to the lips and chin. This can vary in shape and may be concave or convex.

The face shape is made up of straight or curved lines, and sometimes a mixture of the two. Straight line shapes appear angular, chiselled, or firm and solid. They can be triangular, rectangular, square or diamond-shaped. Curved line shapes appear soft, and may be round, oval, pear-shaped or oblong. Shapes which have some straight and some curved lines are defined as heart-shaped or soft square-shaped.

To create a pleasant balance, the hairstyle and face shape need to be compatible. An angular hair cut will not suit a soft rounded face. A soft hair shape will not complement a chiselled face.

Eyes

- Maintain eye contact while you consult your client.
- What colour are your client's eyes?
- What shape are your client's eyes? Do they harmonise with the face shape?
- What are the eyebrows like?
- Does your client wear spectacles?

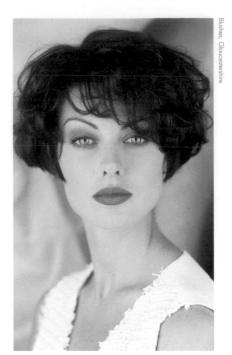

Eye contact is important when you are communicating with your client, as it shows that you are listening to each other. Beware of heavy fringes: they can obstruct eye contact.

Eye colour is a guide to the natural colouring of the client. This is a useful pointer when choosing hair colour.

Eye shape is another element to be considered when choosing which style to create. Ideally, eye, head and face shape should all be complemented by the hairstyle and colour.

The eyebrows frame the eyes. Their shape, size and colour are all significant. A very harsh appearance is created if the eyebrows are removed, and various other effects are created by adding shapely lines. Eyelash and brow tinting help to balance facial effects and give the eyes more definition.

Spectacles should be considered when you are deciding on a hairstyle. Frame and lens colour, size and shape must all be taken into account.

Ears, nose and mouth

- What are the shape, position and size of the client's ears, nose and mouth?
- Do they need covering/disguising or featuring?

Often ears are out of balance, which can affect the cut if you use them as a guide.

Your client may wear a hearing aid, and this may be a sensitive issue. Some clients wish to have all signs of an aid hidden, but others do not mind, and even display it. You should discuss this with your client carefully; she may feel too embarrassed to bring the subject up herself. The size of the aid will need careful consideration when completing the total image.

The position, shape, size and colour of the nose and mouth are very important in the facial expression. The angles that are created can be softening or harsh, and must not be ignored when the image is being planned. Hair shape and make-up can contribute to create the required effect.

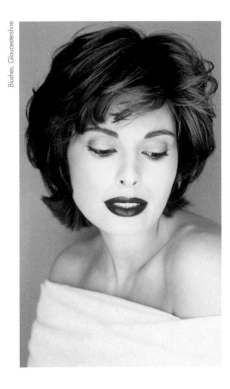

Make-up

- How much make-up is your client wearing?
- What kind of image is she trying to give: natural or glitzy; businesslike or glamorous?

Make-up can enhance features, define eyes, and mask or disguise features or blemishes. How the client uses make-up may give a clue to her personality, dress sense and style.

In business, a well made-up person is seen to be finished, groomed and in control. Without make-up, a person may appear to be 'off duty' or as if she has not made an effort.

Lipstick reflects the colour depth of the skin and eyes, creates light on the face, and defines the lips. Shiny lipstick is most suitable for someone with a glitzy image. Matt lipstick is more suitable for the quieter person, or when a more natural look is required. Lip balm or gloss looks natural and keeps lips soft.

Make-up can create a range of images: soft and kind; bold and extrovert. It can make people feel different about their appearance and so boost confidence if it is properly applied.

Neck and shoulders

- How long or short is your client's neck?
- This will affect the way the hair falls, and so the style chosen.

The length, fullness and width of the neck will affect the fall of the back and nape hair. Longer necks allow better positioning of long hair. They are complemented by high, neat lines – for example, mandarin collars or polo neck tops. Short necks need to be uncluttered, with short hair and low collars.

Hands

- Are the client's hands well groomed?
- Does the client use them to express herself?

We use our hands to communicate too. They are expressive, and the way we look after them is part of the image that we present. Professionals will have polished, groomed nails: manicure will be an essential part of their grooming routine.

The range of colours, polishes and lacquers available allows colour matching with cosmetics, hair colour and clothes. Nail accessories are a new element in hand and nail care.

Body shape

- Straight, angular body shapes can take harder, definite stripes, sculptured or tight lines.
- Rounder shapes can take soft, curved, diffused, relaxed lines.

The body shape needs to be carefully balanced with the amount and size of the hair. A small, clinging hairstyle would look wrong on a large body shape, for example.

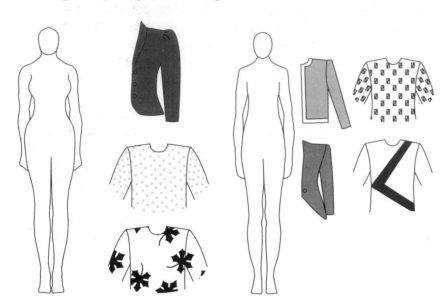

Body shapes
(left) Full
(right) Angular

Lifestyle and personality

How old is your client?
Does she have a hectic lifestyle or career?
What kind of image is she trying to project?
What kind of personality does she have?

Different occasions and lifestyles need to be fitted into our concept of total image. These are as important as the images required to fit certain face or body shapes. Children, teenagers, young couples and older groups all have different hair requirements. Career choice also affects the style we can choose. Receptionists and artists, nurses and bankers all have different lifestyle requirements. Much of this will be discussed during your consultation with the client (see Chapter 3), but do not overlook what she might tell you about her lifestyle during your work with her.

Personality is what makes us individual, and is expressed partly through the way we dress and wear colours, including the colour and style of our hair. When all aspects are right, we achieve a total look which is in focus.

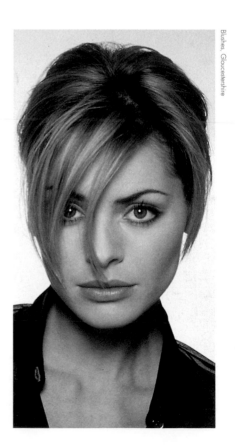

Blushes, Gloucestershire

Colour

☐ Does the client wear 'cool' or 'warm' colours?
☐ Does she wear contrasting or enhancing colours?
☐ What is her natural colouring like: hair, eyes, skin?

Colour influences every part of our lives. We have personal colour – hair, skin, eyes – but we are also surrounded by a colourful environment – landscape, clothes, our surroundings at home and work. Colour affects our perceptions and responses. In nature, colour ranges from the exotic to the subtle. It can be bright or dark, blended or contrasting, soft or muted. The seasons are made up of all kinds of colour and light, from the rich, warm, muted and subdued tones of autumn and winter to the glaring, bright colours of spring and summer.

The choice of colours for dress, hair, skin, eyes, mouth and nails depends on the effects required and the reflection of the colours around us. The basic colours of red, yellow, blue, purple, green and orange are mixed and matched to make an almost endless range. Combinations of colours can be clashing or loud, but others are complementary.

Some colours are warmer or cooler than others. Red and gold are warm; blue and violet are cool. This may be used as a basis for added colour.

Cool	Warm
blue	yellow
pink	orange/copper
red/blue	moss/khaki/green
black	red/orange
white	brown
aqua	cream
bottle green	lime
magenta	peach
burgundy/plum	chestnut
damson/grey	

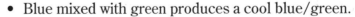

- Blue mixed with green produces a cool blue/green.
- Blue mixed with red produces a cool blue/red.
- Red mixed with orange produces a warm red.
- Green mixed with yellow produces a warm green.
- Black and white are cool colours with blue tones.
- Brown and cream are warm colours with yellow tones.

Some colours are more attractive than other colours: they blend or enhance. These are 'right' colours. Some colours should not be used because they are unsuitable: they clash or fight against or detract from the effects of other colours. These are 'wrong' colours.

Personal, natural colouring is the basis on which to add other colours. Hair, eyes, eyebrows, lashes, lips and skin all have varying depths of colour. This is added to by the light and shade produced by the contours of the face and head. The choice of clothes to be worn – their shape, pattern and colour – all have an

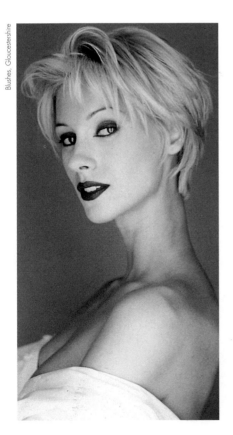

Blushes, Gloucestershire

effect on natural colouring and must be carefully selected for maximum benefit.

We are all attracted to colours that make up our own colouring. Hairdressers should remember this – make sure you don't choose the colours that suit you to use on your client! We are influenced by our friends too: when you shop with a friend, she may encourage you to buy clothes which suit her but not you. The media also influences us, in the colours we choose for our homes, clothes or hair colour.

Choose colours with care. When skin, hair and eye colouring are enhanced by wearing the right colours and tones (warm or cool), we are are close to achieving a total look.

Clothes and accessories

What style of clothing does the client wear: dramatic, relaxed, classic, avant-garde?

What kind of accessories does she wear? Are they understated or extravagant?

Does she have pierced ears?

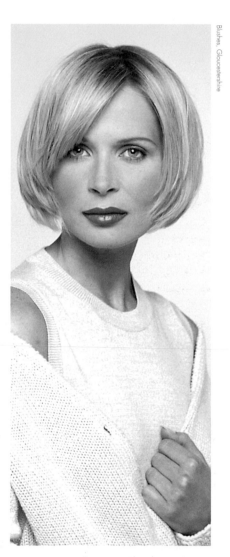

Blushes, Gloucestershire

Your wardrobe says something about the way you run your life. An organised, methodical person may keep her clothes and wardrobe tidy and folded. A disorganised person is more likely not to arrange her wardrobe at all.

The clothes we choose to wear each day reflect the mood we are in. When we feel confident and authoritative, we may want to stand out; when we feel sad and confused, we may want to blend in. What we wear is also indicative of taste and personality. Here are some examples of dress and image:

- *dramatic* – excessive, extreme, demonstrative, eccentric, theatrical, blunt, e.g. Madonna and Paula Yates
- *classic* – traditional, businesslike, formal, groomed, organised, e.g. Princess Diana and Julia Carling
- *romantic* – glamorous, sexy, womanly, shapely, e.g. Marilyn Monroe and Elizabeth Hurley
- *youthful* – neat, cheeky, trendy, fresh-faced, chic, e.g. Kylie Minogue and Zoe Ball
- *pretty* – prim, angelic, feminine, dainty, e.g. Jane Seymour and Helena Bonham-Carter
- *natural* – casual, tousled, relaxed, informal, flexible, e.g. Kim Basinger and Kim Wilde.

Choosing the correct colours means that clothes will mix and match naturally, giving the client lots more to wear. This saves time and money, and gives a feeling of wellbeing and confidence. By asking specific questions, you can develop the skill of linking natural colouring, the colours the client prefers wearing, and the most flattering hair colour. For example:

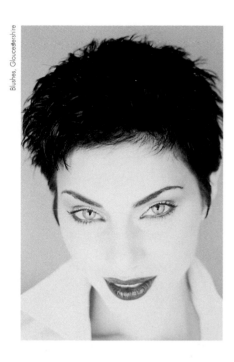

Blushes, Gloucestershire

- What make-up colours do you usually wear?
- Which colours are predominant in your wardrobe?

Are the answers warm or cool colours? If the client is wearing pink lipstick and blusher and black and white clothes, she is giving out a 'cool' message and so would be best with a cool hair tone. If the client is wearing a fuschia pink top and lipstick and tells you that this is her favourite colour, you should dissuade her from choosing chestnut hair colouring.

You will be providing an extra service if your expertise includes suggesting hair colours that will complement the client's choice of make-up and her wardrobe.

Finally, accessories should be in keeping with the total look. They should suit the personality of the wearer and the occasion for which they are to be worn. Earrings can tell us something about the client. Small, neat earrings suggest that the wearer doesn't want to be noticed; flamboyant, theatrical earrings say the opposite. Wearing more than one earring in each ear may be the sign of an extrovert personality.

ASSIGNMENT

With the permission of your manager, carry out a work-based assignment in which you produce a record of your skills in creating a total image. This can comprise sketches and/or photographs, with explanatory notes, for the following processes:
- determining a total look or image
- the use and effect of colour
- the effect that hairstyles have on the face and head shape
- the effect that various accessories have on the hair, face and head
- the effect of make-up and manicure.

After carrying out these practical tasks, write explanatory illustrated notes to show:
1 the steps taken to produce the final effect
2 the variety of techniques used to achieve the desired effect
3 the sources of information used – list the credits
4 details of the client consultation.

You may prefer not to compile sketches, photographs and accompanying notes, but instead to video the assignment and then to give a personal account of what has taken place. Make sure that you address points 1–4 within your account.

QUESTIONS

After completing the assignment, answer these questions in your portfolio.
1 What is a total image or look?
2 What makes one 'look' different from another?
3 What are the effects of shape and colour?
4 How can the use of clothes and accessories affect the total image?

5 What are the features of currently fashionable looks?
6 Apart from the use of books, magazines, periodicals, film and photography, what other sources of inspiration can you list?

CHAPTER 3

Professional consultation

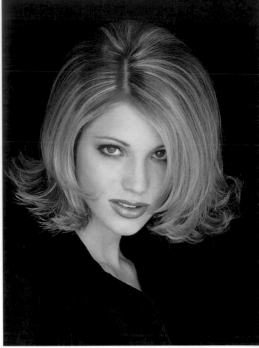

Mark Hill for Wella

INTRODUCTION

Professional consultation undertaken by experienced staff is a valuable process which follows a specific sequence of events. Sometimes consultation is used as a stand-alone service; at other times it is combined with pre-booked services and treatments. In either situation, this service provides the most important form of communication between salon staff and the client. It is used to find out information, to give professional advice, to choose a course of action, and to identify opportunities for sales.

The ideal consultation process is one where there is an exchange of information between client and stylist which will enable a suitable and successful course of action to be taken. It is intended to closely examine the client's needs and requirements. This includes listening and carefully considering clients' requests.

The way in which questions are asked is important. 'Closed' questions, i.e. those that require a simple yes or no answer, provide minimal information and therefore should be avoided. It is better to use an 'open' questioning style – How? Why? When? Where? The more information that can be gained, the more satisfactory consultation is likely to be. It needs to be carefully weighed and considered. If this does not happen, serious mistakes can happen and the client will be dissatisfied.

THE PURPOSE OF CONSULTATION

For the client

Consultation gives the client an advisory service which is linked to the variety of treatments and services a salon may provide. The consultation process helps to determine the client's needs based on lifestyle, personal preferences and style suitability. Other aspects, for example manageability and aftercare, should be addressed during the process.

For the stylist

Consultation lets the stylist make a series of professional judgements. These provide the basis for planning the right course of action. The outcome should be beneficial to both the client and the stylist. This is the most effective sales tool that a salon can provide.

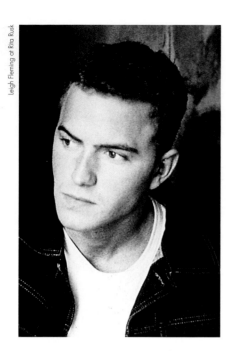

Leigh Fleming at Rita Rusk

THE CONSULTATION PROCESS

This should follow a logical sequence of events, which will start with the reception of a client. It will lead on to either booking an appointment or carrying out technical services for the client. The variety of aspects within professional consultation are illustrated in this chapter using building blocks. The sequence in which they are found here is not necessarily the only order in which they should be used. However, all the blocks together cover all the important aspects of consultation.

Reception

Personal information

Why us?

Client expectations

Lifestyle

Physical features

Character and personality

Age

Hair constraints

Manageability

Cost implications

Reception of clients

The reception of clients should include:

- listening carefully
- giving your undivided attention
- giving an immediate response and acknowledgement
- displaying the correct posture and body language
- providing adequate time for the client.

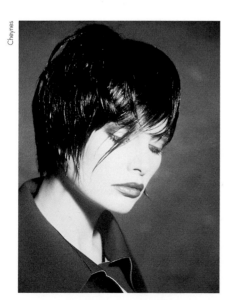

Cheynes

From a psychological point of view, we have about ten seconds from the first eye contact to convey the right professional image. The client will consciously or subconsciously analyse what she sees. Therefore, our appearance is as important as our expression. Is our body language welcoming? Are we maintaining a professional level of communication? You should never appear familiar or authoritative with new potential clients.

After the first few seconds, direct your client to a quieter area of the salon. Remember that a personal consultation should remain personal, private and *confidential*.

Personal information

- Carefully record the client's personal details: name, address, telephone number, fax number and so on.
- Note any particular requests: product, process, particular shampoos or colours.
- Check the stock to make sure that you have the right materials, and put them on one side with the client's name on them so that they won't get used up before the appointment.
- The need for confidentiality is important and must always be strictly observed.
- Retain all relevant information for future use in consultations.

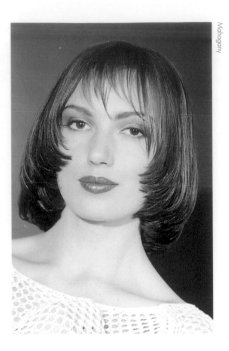
Mahogany

Position yourself opposite your client, not next to her, or behind her looking in a mirror. Your eyes should be level with or slightly lower than your client's. If you have specific records to complete, explain exactly what purpose they have. If you are open with your client in this way, she will feel comfortable and this will aid the flow of information.

Why us?

How did the client find out about your salon?

Was it a personal recommendation?
Was she attracted by the salon's comfort, high standard of hygiene, or services offered?
Was she attracted by another client's style?
Did she respond to an advert, presentation or promotion?
Was she attracted by the salon appearance, window displays or design?
Was it a casual visit?

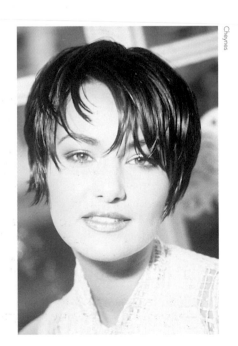
Cheynes

It is valuable to find out why the potential client has come to your salon, so that you can monitor new business. It would be very unprofessional to ask where the client has had her hair done in the past, but if she offers this information, that is a different matter.

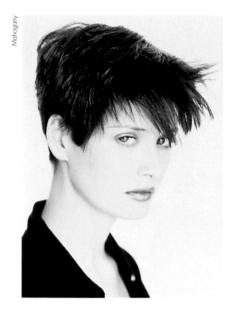
Mahogany

Client expectations

☐ Does the client have something specific in mind?
☐ How was the style/image selected? What is required and necessary?
☐ Does this conflict with the client's expectations? Discuss techniques, products and effects with the client.
☐ Examine the client's hair and scalp. Determine the tests required and diagnose any scalp or hair conditions (see pages 26–35).
☐ Determine the need for referral to a senior member of staff or a doctor.
☐ Note any photographs or pictures brought as illustrations by the client, and retain them.
☐ Interpret the client's request.

Does the client want the hair cut, dressed, coloured or the volume increased? Has she a specific treatment or style in mind? Does she have any examples of it? These are all essential questions that must be asked before any suitability analysis can take place. You need direction and a place to start from. Do you have any examples of hairstyles to show the client if she hasn't brought any? When you have reached the point where you have a range of options, you can decide which are suitable.

Lifestyle

Bear the following factors in mind when deciding on a suitable style:

☐ client's social and leisure pursuits, general activities
☐ fashion needs, special occasions
☐ age: different styles are favoured by various age groups
☐ work aspects: job requirements/interviews/communications
☐ existing wardrobe
☐ looks required.

Remember that people are constrained by what they do for a living or what they like to do in their spare time. Usually, people who work in environments where they have face-to-face contact with clients have to be more particular about the image they portray. This is a very important factor in style selection.

From a leisure point of view, you should consider whether the client does a lot of sport or exercise. If so, the hairstyle will have to be versatile and able to withstand a lot of washing. Also, think about how the style could be handled to create a number of different effects when the client is going out.

You could choose one of the following 'looks':

- *classic* – timeless appeal
- *fashionable* – currently in vogue

- *avant-garde* – ahead of fashion
- *commercial* – mass market appeal
- *fantasy* – extreme, imaginative, theme-based
- *high fashion (haute coiffure)* – the very latest trends
- *allegorical* – theme- or fantasy-based styles
- *historical* – depicting an event or period of time
- *original* – usually individual, adapted styles.

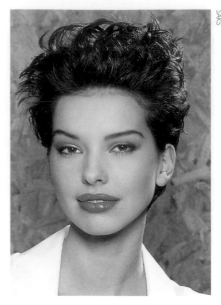

If you are styling for a special occasion, it is worth asking what dress will be worn. A beautiful gown needs to be accompanied by an elegant hairstyle. However, this style will need to be altered for normal wear.

- Many clients want practical and manageable styles for work.
- Nurses, doctors and caterers, among others, may require styles which keep the hair off the face, or they may have to wear face and head coverings at work.
- Dancers, athletes and skaters, among others, need hairstyles which will not get in their eyes and obscure their vision.
- Fashion models may require elaborate styles for special photographic or modelling sessions or displays.

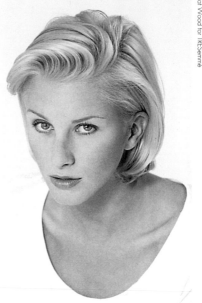

Physical features

Remember to note and consider the following when choosing a style for your client:

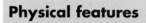

- hair length, perimeter shape, volume, weight distribution and direction
- body size and proportions
- prominent facial features and bone structure
- balance and overall symmetry
- profile and head shape
- skin tone and colour
- glasses and hearing aids.

These aspects have been discussed in Chapters 1 and 2. Remember, the outline of the client's face is unique and it must be complemented by the style. The style can be used to diminish or exaggerate the face shape.

- Square and oblong face shapes are made more prominent by sleek, flat styles, and diminished by fuller sides.
- Large round faces look rounder with full hair, but longer with the hair dressed higher.
- Hard jaw lines stand out more when the hair is dressed back, but appear softer with it directed forwards.

The features of the face can also be disguised or enhanced by the style you choose.

- A prominent nose may be reduced by angling the hair at the front or by avoiding central partings.

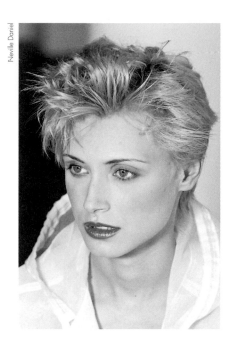

- Protruding ears should be covered up. Remember to leave enough length when cutting.
- Double or prominent chins are exposed by sweeping hair movements.
- Eye wrinkles are made more obvious by straight line shapes. Angling the hair away from them can soften them.
- Low, high, wide or narrow foreheads may be disguised by angling the front hair and varying the fringe position.
- Hearing aids may need to be covered. Sufficient hair length needs to be left while cutting to do this.

Personality

Is your client:

- [ ] confident and outgoing
- [ ] shy, timid and retiring
- [ ] professional and businesslike
- [ ] happy, smiling and pleasant
- [ ] dour, sullen and despondent?

Character and personality can often override physical features when you are choosing a style for your client. A self-confident client will be able to wear looks that a self-conscious client cannot. Make sure you take this into account so that mistakes are not made.

Age

- [ ] What age group is your client in?
- [ ] What style might she want?

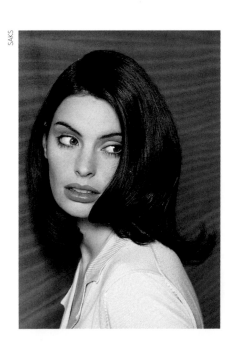

The following guidelines commonly apply:

- *child* – simple, practical shapes
- *teenager* – something slightly different, especially from older styles
- *young married* – something suitable for work, attractive styles
- *parent* – practical and attractive styles, often shorter styles
- *middle aged* – softening shapes to disguise wrinkles
- *senior citizen* – softening shapes
- *young businessmen* – fashionable cuts
- *older men* – simple, practical styles.

You should note this, but remember we live in a community that is progressive, which can throw off convention and which welcomes visual change.

Hair constraints

Consider the following hair constraints when selecting the style:

- ☐ amount and distribution
- ☐ texture, type and condition
- ☐ previous treatment
- ☐ movement and growth patterns.

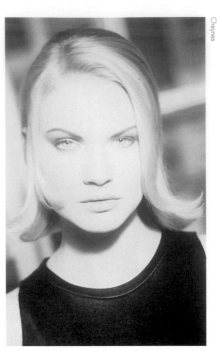

Cheynes

Make sure you analyse the hair and scalp adequately so that you only present suitable options to the client. Specific hair tests are discussed later in the chapter (pages 26–8). The following guidelines might help:

- Hair in poor condition seldom looks right and is difficult to style. The condition will need to be corrected before cutting takes place. Healthy shining hair contributes to good cutting.
- Fine, thin hair requires careful attention and cutting techniques that make it appear thicker. Avoid extreme tapering, thinning and texturising; instead, for the best results use club cutting on this type of hair. Very fine, limp hair soon loses its shape. Aids such as thickeners or mousse may be used to enhance the cut shape.
- Dry, thick hair may require cutting techniques that will allow the hair to be styled sleek and smooth. All forms of texturising are useful with this hair type.
- Coarse hair may require containment so that it does not appear too heavy and awkward. Tapering, thinning and castle serrations can be helpful.

Always look at the client's natural hair growth patterns too, as these will affect any style chosen.

Manageability

Consider the following manageability issues:

- ☐ time available for client to style hair
- ☐ ease of styling hair
- ☐ client's ability to style hair
- ☐ how frequently client washes hair
- ☐ which products should be used at home.

Different styles need different amounts of commitment from the client once she leaves the salon. You must take these into account when consulting with the client to make sure that she will carry on being happy with the style you both choose until it is time for her next appointment.

Cost implications

☐ Which techniques do you intend to use?
☐ What does your style require in terms of time and products?

When a suitable course of action is determined, the client should then be made aware of all the costs for services and treatments involved.

AFTER THE CONSULTATION

Style or service selection

You and the client will select the required style or service together. To avoid disappointment, you must ensure that she knows exactly what is entailed, what it will cost and how long it will take.

- Listen carefully to what is requested.
- Communicate the possible effects.
- Explain why certain effects are not possible.
- Give good reasons for suggested actions.
- Ensure that the client understands what is being said.
- Agree on a final and suitable course of action.
- Assure and reassure throughout.
- Make it clear if follow-up appointments are necessary.

Achievement of agreed effects

- Carry out the technical actions.
- Ensure that the actions are those agreed and intended.
- Ensure that future appointments are made on completion of the work.
- Manage the client's safety and goodwill throughout.
- Record the client's satisfaction.

Problems arising

If the final effects are not what was thought to have been agreed, the client may make a complaint.

- Listen carefully to the client's complaint.
- Resolve the problem immediately or as soon as possible.
- Do not allow the disagreement to affect the salon environment, and act sensibly and with decorum at all times.
- Record the complaint.
- Refer to senior staff if necessary.
- Refer to the management so that they can inform the insurers if necessary.
- If the client is not happy, she may want to take legal action. This must be dealt with by the management.

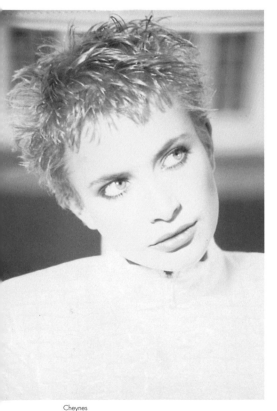

Cheynes

HAIR AND SKIN TESTS

To minimise the likelihood of problems arising, there are various tests you can carry out to help you diagnose the condition and likely reaction of your client's hair and skin. These tests will help you decide what actions to take before, during or after the application of hairdressing processes. Remember to record all results on to the client's record card.

Skin test

A skin test (also known as a predisposition test, patch test, Sabouraud-Rousseau test or hypersensitivity test) is used to assess the reaction of the skin to chemicals or chemical products. In the salon it is mainly used before tinting. Some people are allergic to external contact of chemicals, e.g. dermatitis due to tinting. Some are allergic to irritants reacting internally, e.g. asthma and hay fever. Others may be allergic to both internal and external irritants.

To find out whether a client's skin reacts to chemicals in permanent tints, carry out the following test:

1 Mix a little tint to be used with the correct amount of hydrogen peroxide – as recommended by the maker.
2 Clean an area of skin about 8 mm square, behind the ear or in the arm fold. Use spirit on cottonwool to remove the grease from the skin.
3 Apply a little of the tint mixture to the skin.
4 Allow it to dry.
5 Cover the tint patch with collodion to protect it. Ask your client to report any discomfort or irritation that occurs over the next 24–48 hours. Arrange to see your client at the end of this time so that you can check for signs of reaction.
6 If there is a positive response – any skin reaction, such as inflammation, soreness, swelling, irritation or discomfort – do not use this colouring treatment. Never ignore the result of a skin test. If a skin test showed a reaction and you carried on anyway, there might be a much more serious reaction: this might affect the whole body and could, for example, lead to dermatitis.
7 If there is a negative response – no reaction – you can carry out the treatment proposed.

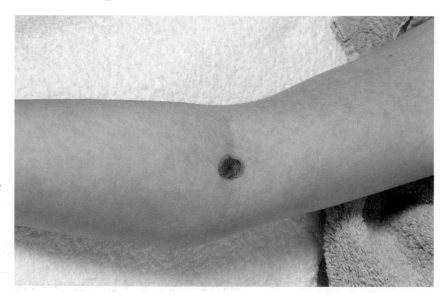

Skin test

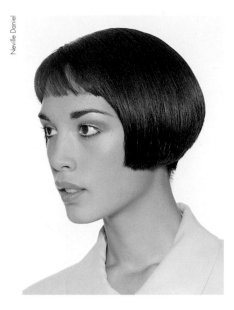

Neville Daniel

Strand test

A strand test or hair strand colour test is used to assess the resultant colour on a strand or section of hair after colour has been processed and developed. It is carried out as follows:

1 Most colouring products just require the time recommended by the manufacturer – check their instructions.
2 Rub a strand of hair lightly with a paper tissue or the back of a comb to remove the surplus tint.
3 Check whether the colour remaining is evenly distributed throughout the hair's length. If it is even, remove the rest of the tint. If it is uneven, allow processing to continue, if necessary applying more tint. If any of the hair on the head is not being treated, you can compare the evenness of colour in the tinted hair with that in the untinted hair.

Colour test

This test is used to assess the suitability of a chosen colour, the amount of processing time that will be required, and the final colour that will result. Apply the tint or bleaching products you propose to use to a cutting of the client's hair and process as recommended.

Test cutting

In this test, a piece of hair cut from the head is processed to check its suitability, the amount of processing required and the timing, before the process is carried out. The test is used for colouring, straightening, relaxing, reducing synthetic colouring, bleaching and incompatibility.

Test curl

This test is made on the hair to determine the lotion suitability, the strength, the curler size, the timing of processing and the development. It is used before perming.

Curl check or test

This test is used to assess the development of curl in the perming process. The test is used periodically throughout a perm and for final assessment of the result.

'Peroxide' test

This test is made on hair that has been decoloured or stripped of its synthetic colour. The test is used to assess the effectiveness of the process and to check that no synthetic pigment remains. Any synthetic colour remaining will oxidise later and darken again within two or three days. If the hair darkens after testing, remove all the chemicals from the test section, then reapply the decolourant. It may take several applications to strip all of the unwanted colour.

Incompatibility test

Perm lotions and other chemicals applied to the hair may react with chemicals that have already been used, such as home-use products. The incompatibility test is therefore used to detect chemicals which could react with hairdressing processes such as colouring and perming. It is carried out as follows:

1 Protect your hands by wearing gloves.
2 Place a small cutting of hair in a small dish.
3 Pour a mixture of hydrogen peroxide and ammonium hydroxide on to the hair. Make sure that you are not bending over the dish, to avoid splashing the chemicals on to your face.
4 Watch for signs of bubbling, heating or discolouration. These indicate that the hair already contains incompatible chemicals. The hair should not be permed, tinted or bleached if there are any signs of reaction. Perming treatment might discolour or break the hair, and could burn the skin.

Elasticity test

This test is used to determine how much the hair will stretch and then return to its original position – an indicator of its condition. By taking a hair between the fingers and stretching it you can assess the amount of spring it has. If the hair breaks easily, care needs to be taken before applying any hairdressing process and further tests are indicated – a test curl or a test cutting, for example. Natural healthy hair in good condition will be elastic and more likely to retain the effects of physical curling, setting or blow shaping longer. It will also take chemical processes more readily. Hair with little elasticity will not hold physical shaping or chemical processes satisfactorily.

Porosity test

This test is used to assess the ability of the hair to absorb moisture or liquids – another indicator of condition. If the cuticle is torn or broken, it will soon lose its moisture and become dry. It may be able to absorb liquids quicker, but its ability to retain them is reduced. If the cuticle is smooth, unbroken and tightly packed, it may resist the passage of moisture or liquids. By running the fingertips through the hair, from points to roots, you can assess the degree of roughness. The rougher the hair, the more porous it will be and the faster it will absorb chemicals.

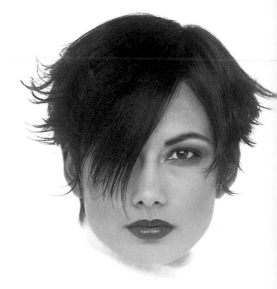

Cheynes

HAIR AND SCALP DISEASES, CONDITIONS AND DEFECTS

Diseases of the hair and scalp may be caused by a variety of infectious organisms. Signs or symptoms are presented which enable us to recognise them. Initial examination, during consultation, should be carried out before any hairdressing procedure is applied. If this precaution is not taken, there is a danger of cross-infection where both hairdresser and clients may contract and spread disease. Other hair and scalp *conditions* or *defects* may be due to abnormal formation or the result of a variety of chemical and physical causes. They are not infectious.

Bacterial infectious diseases

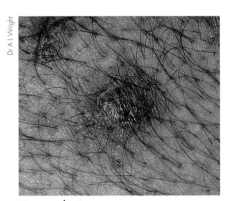

Furunculosis

- **Furunculosis** Boils or abcesses.
  Cause An infection of the hair follicles by staphylococcal bacteria.
  Symptoms Raised, inflamed, pus-filled spots; irritation, swelling and pain.
  Treatment By a doctor.

- **Sycosis** A bacterial infection of the hairy parts of the face.
  Cause Bacteria attack the upper part of the hair follicle, spreading to the lower follicle.
  Symptoms Small, yellow spots around the follicle mouth; burning, irritation and general inflammation.
  Treatment By a doctor.

- **Impetigo** A bacterial infection of the upper skin layers.
  Cause Staphylococcal or streptococcal infection.
  Symptoms First, a burning sensation; small spots appear and become dry; honey-coloured crusts form; spots merge to form larger areas.
  Treatment Antibiotics, given by a doctor.

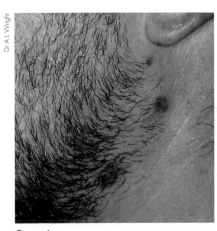

Sycosis

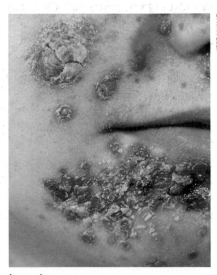

Impetigo

- **Folliculitis** Inflammation of the hair follicles.
  Cause A bacterial infection, or due to chemical action
  (e.g. careless application of CPW lotions) or physical action
  (e.g. shaving or scratching).
  Symptoms Inflamed follicles.
  Treatment By a doctor.

Viral infectious diseases

- **Herpes simplex (cold sore)** A viral infection of the skin.
  Cause Possibly exposure to extreme heat or cold, or a
  reaction to food or drugs; the skin may carry the virus for
  years without exhibiting any symptoms.
  Symptoms Burning, irritation, swelling and inflammation
  precede the appearance of fluid-filled blisters, usually on the
  lips and surrounding areas.
  Treatment By a doctor, if serious, or with products from a
  chemist.

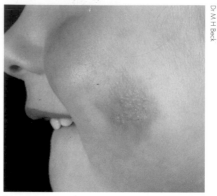

Herpes simplex

- **Herpes zoster (shingles)** A viral infection of the epidermis
  and nerve endings.
  Cause Possibly due to chicken pox in earlier years – the virus
  may have lain dormant in the skin.
  Symptoms Painful blisters appear, often on one side only of
  the head or body; sore inflamed areas result. This may be
  preceded by fever. Aching and pain may continue after the
  condition has cleared.
  Treatment By a doctor.

- **Influenza** and the **common cold** Viral infections of the body.
  Cause Viruses attacking the cells of the body.
  Symptoms Fever, sneezing, aching, streaming nose, etc.
  Treatment By a doctor, if serious, or with cold-relief remedies
  from a chemist.

- **Verrucae (warts)** A viral infection of the skin.
  Cause The lower epidermis is attacked by the virus, which
  causes the skin to harden and skin cells to multiply.
  Symptoms Raised, roughened skin, often brown or
  discoloured. There may be irritation and soreness. Warts are
  common on the hands and face.
  Treatment By a doctor.

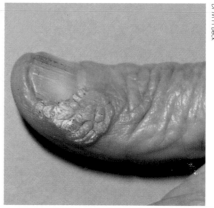

A wart

Fungal infectious diseases

- **Tinea capitis** Ringworm of the head.
  Cause Fungal infection of the skin or hair.
  Symptoms Circular bald areas of grey or whitish skin,
  surrounded by red, active rings; hairs broken close to the
  skin, which looks dull and rough. The fungus lives off the
  keratin in the skin and hair. This disease is common in
  children.
  Treatment By a doctor.

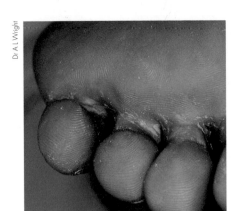

Tinea pedis

- **Tinea pedis (athlete's foot)** Ringworm of the feet.
  Cause Fungal infection of the skin between the toes, which becomes soft and soggy. The disease is common among people who use swimming pools or do not dry their feet thoroughly, and those standing for long periods (including hairdressers).
  Symptoms Soft, sore skin; sometimes bleeding; a bad odour; some irritation.
  Treatment By a doctor or with products from a chemist.

Infectious diseases caused by animal parasites

- **Scabies** A skin reaction to the itch mite.
  Cause A tiny animal mite – *Sarcoptes scabiei* – which burrows under the skin, where it lays its eggs.
  Symptoms Reddish spots and greyish burrow lines over all parts of the body, particularly in the skin folds between the fingers and toes. The disease causes intense irritation due to the parasitic activities under the skin. It is rarely found on the face or scalp.
  Treatment By a doctor.

- **Pediculosis capitis** Infestation of the head by lice.
  Cause The animal parasite – *Pediculus humanus capitis* – attacks the skin and feeds by puncturing the skin to suck the blood; it lays its eggs (ova) on the hair, close to the skin.
  Symptoms Irritation; red scratch marks; the presence of lice or eggs at the back of the head and ears. Lice are unable to jump, but are easily spread by direct contact.
  Treatment By a doctor or with special products from a chemist. Not to be treated in the salon.

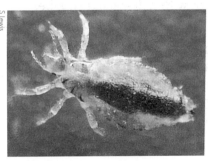

A head louse

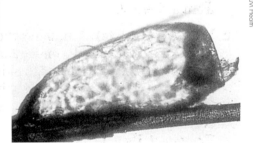

A louse egg (nit)

- **Pulex irritans (human flea)** Infestation of human-feeding fleas.
  Cause The animal parasite – the flea – is wingless but able to jump from one host to another. It feeds on human blood after biting the skin and lays its eggs off the host, usually in carpets, dust cracks, clothing or bedding.
  Symptoms The bite causes bright red spots, surrounded by a pink patch, and irritation.
  Treatment Hoovering, dusting, cleaning of clothes and bed.

Non-infectious conditions of the skin and hair

- **Alopecia** Hair loss or baldness. There are several distinct patterns or types:

  Alopecia areata is the name given to baldness in circular areas. It is common on the scalp. These areas may eventually join to form **alopecia totalis**, complete loss of hair from the scalp, or **alopecia capitis**, complete baldness of the head.

  Alopecia universalis is complete baldness of the body.

  Male pattern alopecia is the most common form of hair loss. Hair recedes at the temples, spreading to the top of the scalp. The rate of progression varies individually. It is common in the late teenage years of men and the later years of women. Its cause is hereditary, but androgen hormone levels and age contribute.

  Premature alopecia is hair loss, thinning and baldness in the early years of men.

  Alopecia cicatrical is the term given to the loss of hair follicles and subsequent hair growth due to skin scarring.

  Alopecia traction is the loss of hair due to excessive pulling, e.g. plucking, rolling, tonging, brushing and hair straightening.

  Cause The hair follicles are unable to produce new hairs to replace the old ones. This may be attributed to the malfunction of hair growth mechanisms in the hair papilla and germinal matrix and variation of the anagen, telogen and catagen hair growth patterns. Other factors include general health, diet, age, sex, heredity, climate, hormone distribution, stress and the effects of a variety of physical and chemical treatments.

  Symptoms These vary according to the type of alopecia exhibited, but may manifest as diffuse thinning hair, small or large areas of hair loss, or completely denuded scalp or skin.

  Treatment There are a variety of treatments prescribed by doctors, trichologists and hairdressers, with varying effectiveness. There is no known cure for baldness or alopecia as yet, with the exception of traction alopecia which may be self-inflicted or due to physical ill-treatment.

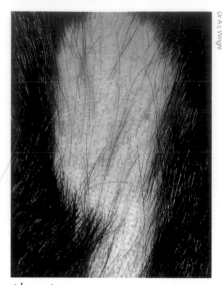

Alopecia areata

- **Acne** A disorder of the hair follicles and sebaceous glands.

  Cause Increased sebum and other matter blocks the hair follicle; the skin reacts to this blockage as though it were a foreign body such as a splinter.

  Symptoms Raised spots or bumps in the skin, commonly on the face and forehead; soreness, irritation and inflammation; severe cases produce cysts and scarring.

  Treatment By a doctor.

- **Eczema/dermatitis** At its simplest, red inflamed skin.

  Cause There are several causes, with either internal or external factors; it may be due to physical irritation or to an allergic response of the skin.

  Symptoms These range from slightly inflamed areas of skin to severe splitting and weeping areas; there may be irritation,

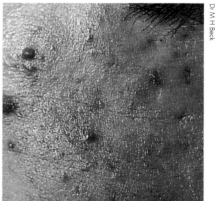

Acne

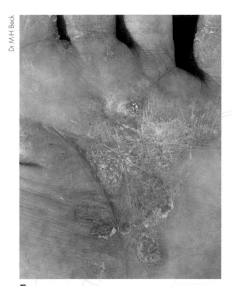

Eczema

soreness and pain; in advanced stages the underlying skin may become infected.
Treatment By a doctor.

■ **Pityriasis capitis (dandruff)** Dry, scaling scalp.
Cause Overproduction of skin cells due to physical or chemical irritants and possibly aggravated by fungal infection.
Symptoms Small, very fine, white, loose scales of skin. These may irritate the scalp to varying degrees; they are also unsightly when they fall on to shoulders, and may cause the sufferer some anxiety. If the scales stick to the skin, small patches of dry skin result; this can cause inflammation. If the scales become moist and greasy, they stick to the skin and the condition known as **scurf** results. Dandruff can be accompanied by **conjunctivitis**, eye inflammation, or **blepharitis**, eyelid inflammation.
Treatment By various anti-dandruff medicines and shampoos. The condition is often treated at home. Refer serious cases to a doctor or trichologist.

■ **Seborrhoea** Excessive greasiness of the hair and skin.
Cause Overproduction of sebum which may be due to chemical or physical irritants, e.g. overstimulation by combing, brushing or massage. Use of greasy or oily products adds to the problem.
Symptoms Very greasy, lank hair and greasy skin, which make grooming and dressing of the hair difficult.
Treatment Regular washing with suitable shampoos; reduce physical or chemical stimulation; application of special anti-grease treatments. Serious conditions should be referred to a doctor or trichologist.

■ **Psoriasis** An inflamed, abnormal thickening of the skin.
Cause Unknown.
Symptoms Areas of thickened skin, which may be raised and circular; silvery or yellow scaling may be present; the skin may be very sore, itchy or painful.
Treatment By a doctor or dermatologist.

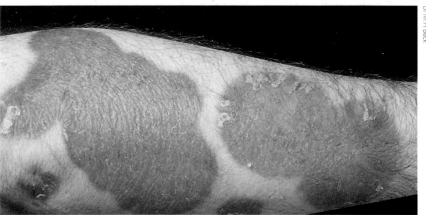

Psoriasis

Defects of the hair

- **Fragilitas crinium (split ends)** Fragile, poorly conditioned hair.
  Cause Harsh physical or chemical treatments, particularly some hairdressing processes; effects of weather (sun, wind, frost); extremes of climate (hot, cold, dry); exposure to sea (salt, sand); effects of chlorine in swimming pools.
  Symptoms Dry, splitting hair ends; the hair may be very coarse and rough.
  Treatment Cutting the hair ends; conditioning; application of substantive conditioners or restructurants.

- **Damaged cuticle** Broken, split, torn hair.
  Cause Harsh physical or chemical treatments.
  Symptoms Rough, raised, missing areas of cuticle; hair loses its moisture and becomes dry and porous.
  Treatment Application of rehabilitating creams, moisturisers, restructurants or protein hydrolysates.

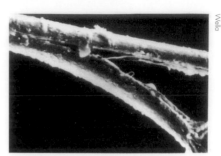

Fragilitas crinium

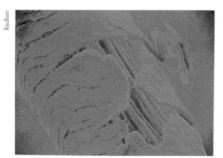

A damaged hair cuticle

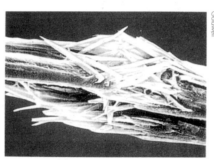

Damaged hair

- **Trichorrhexis nodosa** Nodules on the hair shaft, containing splitting sections of hair.
  Cause Harsh physical or chemical treatments.
  Symptoms Areas of swelling nodules and lengthwise splitting of the hair.
  Treatment Cutting the hair ends and conditioning with hair thickeners may help.

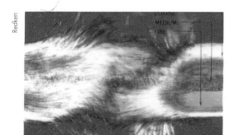

Trichorrhexis nodosa

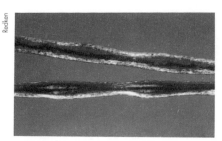
Monilethrix

- **Monilethrix** Beaded hair.
  Cause Irregular development of the hair when forming in the follicle, aggravated by harsh chemical and physical treatments.
  Symptoms Beadlike swellings and constrictions of the hair shafts; hair often breaks close to the skin; there may be small or large areas of short broken hair.
  Treatment By a doctor; general hair care and conditioning may help.

- **Canities** Grey hair or a mixture of hair colour.
  Cause Irregular functioning of the colour pigment formation mechanism during hair growth; white hair occurs in the absence of normal hair colour pigmentation.
  Symptoms The presence of white hairs in small or large areas.
  Treatment Application of synthetic colourings, e.g. tinting.

- **Ringed hair** Alternating rings of white and coloured hair – a form of canities.
  Cause Irregular distribution of pigment during hair formation or regeneration.
  Symptoms Distinct bands of coloured and colourless hair.
  Treatment There are few effective treatments other than hair colouring.

- **Albinism** A congenital colouring defect affecting the eyes, hair and skin. **Partial albinism** occurs when the amount of pigment varies; **total albinism** occurs when the pigment is totally absent.
  Cause An imbalance or total absence of melanin production or distribution throughout the body.
  Symptoms Eyes appear pink due to lack of pigment; hair may be white in small or large areas; skin may have white patches or be very pale.
  Treatment By a doctor.

- **Sebaceous cyst** Swelling of a sebaceous gland.
  Cause The gland becomes blocked, possibly due to a growth of cells from the gland wall.
  Symptoms Bumps, lumps or swellings, 15–20 mm across, on the scalp; they are soft to the touch due to their fluid sebum content.
  Treatment Removal of the cyst and its contents by a doctor.

ASSIGNMENT

With the permission of your manager, devise a consultation system to meet the needs of your salon and its staff. The system could take the form of a questionnaire and/or checklist. It could provide for the salon:

- a comprehensive system of consultation
- an effective system for recording client consultations.

The system should be able to:

- identify customer requirements
- cover all the salon's services, treatments and products
- provide up-to-date customer records
- record professional advice and recommendations
- record the results of any hair and skin tests.

In order to provide a comprehensive system capable of being used by you and other staff, you must take into account the many factors that influence decision-making, such as age, head and facial shapes, hair and scalp analysis, and hair growth patterns.

Remember to keep examples of your system in use, for your portfolio.

QUESTIONS

After completing the assignment, answer these questions in your portfolio.

1 Why is consultation necessary? List the questions that you would use.

2 Why is communication vital? Note down the different ways of communicating with your clients.

3 What is the importance of recording information? List the ways in which this can be done.

4 Describe the different aspects of non-verbal communication.

5 With reference to role-play, describe different methods of consultation.

CHAPTER 4

Creative cutting

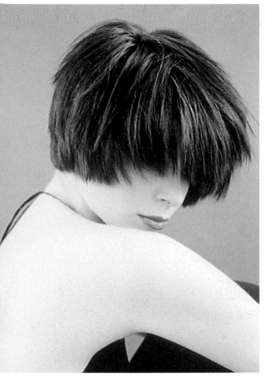

Charles Worthington

INTRODUCTION

The design and construction of fashionable hair shapes should always be carefully considered. You should think through the technique and application. Remember that your cut is the foundation on which all other hairdressing rests.

Creative design is deciding what needs to be done, making the right choices and selecting what will suit the client and her requirements. It is essential that you and your client understand each other: what is referred to as short, long or medium needs to be mutually agreed. To assume you are both thinking of the same length could be disastrous for the satisfactory completion of your total image.

Always make sure you have enough time for the cutting process. Nothing is achieved by rushing work – other than bad habits.

Cutting and styling are intrinsic to the final look. Within this chapter we provide step-by-step guidance to cutting designs, as well as relevant background information. The building blocks you need to consider include:

Shape and form

Lines and angles

Adopted techniques

Apparent texture

Movement and direction

Dimensions, distribution and abundance

Colour depth and tone

Condition

Hair type

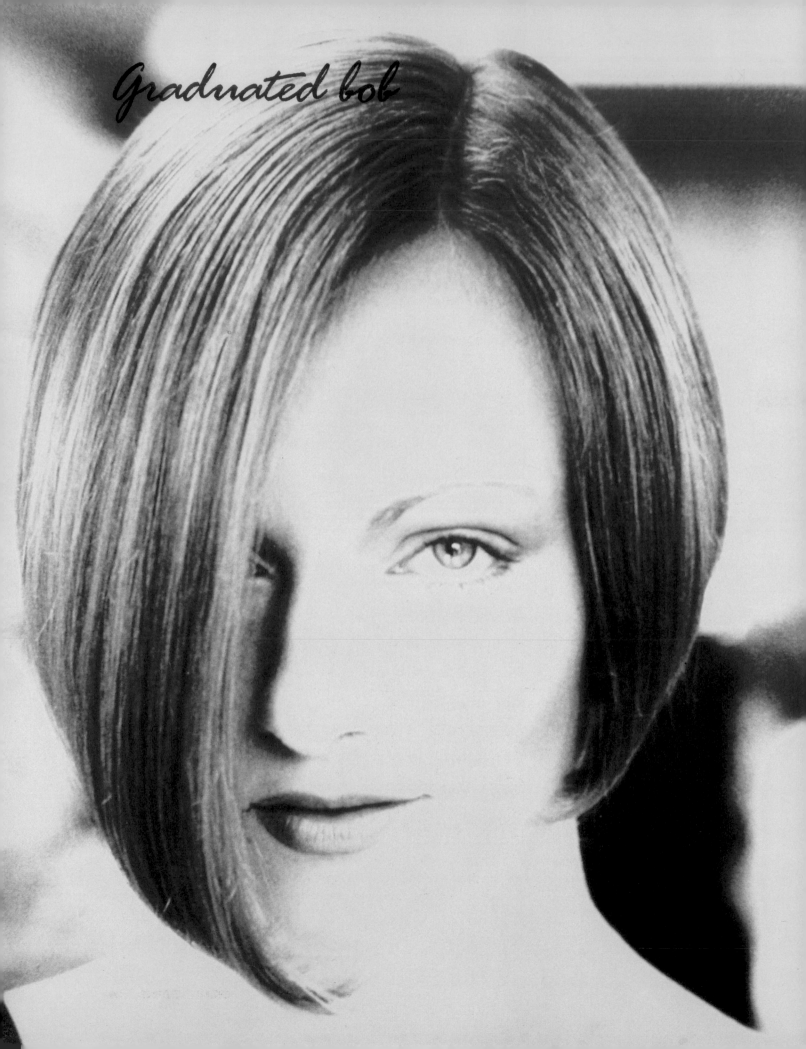

Graduated bob

Key building blocks

Shape and form

The asymmetrical effect is achieved by the low side parting. The smooth hair finishes the overall effect.

Lines and angles

The cleanly cut inverted 'V' shaped sides enable the hair to cling to the head. The angle of the hair terminates with weight towards the front.

Movement and direction

All the hair is directed into a sleek, smooth, flattering shape.

Dimensions

These are not exaggerated, but softly complement the facial features.

Colour depth and tone

The coloured regions contrast with the surrounding hair which gives emphasis to the hair line and direction.

Step-by-step guidance

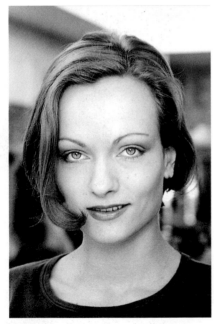

1 The client before the haircut.

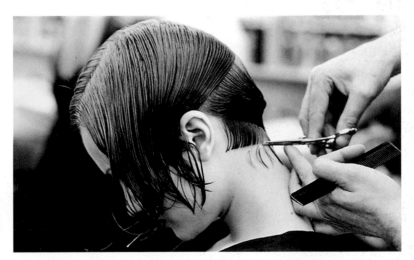

2 After shampooing and conditioning, take the first section from the lower occipital bone, ear to ear. Cut it flat on to the skin, then graduate it at the sides.

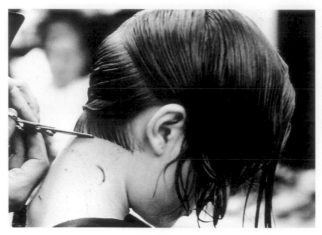

3 Repeat this on the other side.

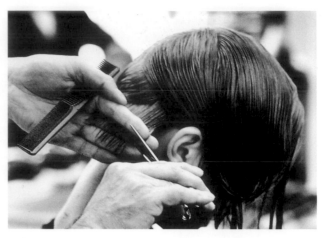

4 Elevate the remainder of the section by 45° to achieve regular graduation.

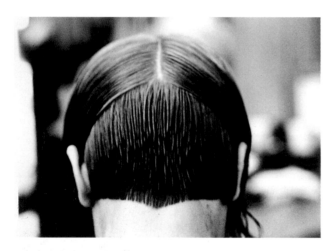

5 The completed back section.

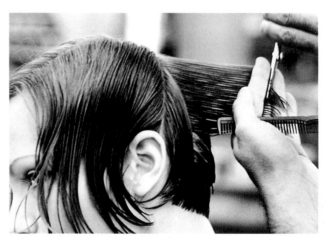

6 Section the hair from the top of the crown to behind the ear and cut it vertically.

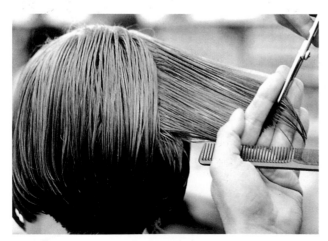

7 Continue this all around the head.

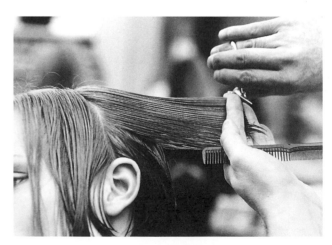

8 Direct the hair back off the face to ensure that the right amount of length will be left at the jawline.

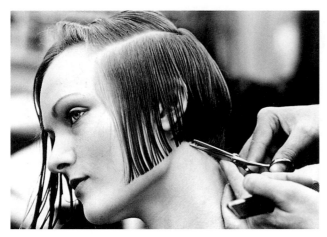

9 Then cut it freehand behind the ear to accentuate the angle. Direct the hair backwards from the chin to create maximum length at the front and cut using tension to accentuate the angle along the jawline.

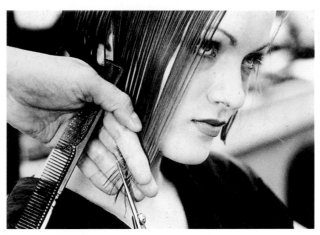

10 Repeat this on the other side.

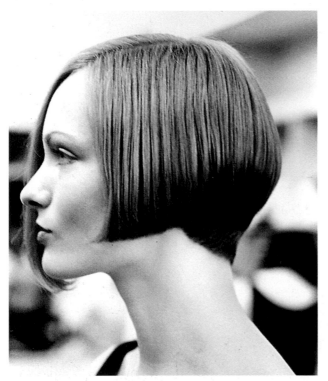

11 The finished left side.

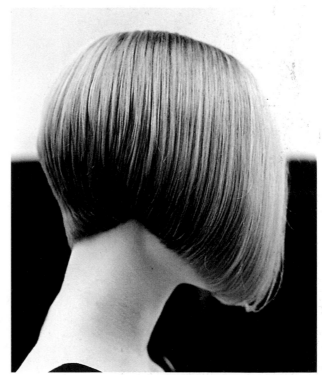

12 The finished right side. The hair has been blow dried using a round brush and styling lotion, then sleeked with wax.

Short contemporary graduation

Key building blocks

Shape and form

The volumised raised crown counterbalances the width and depth of the forehead. Attractive small ears are enhanced, even accentuated, by tucked hair. Cheek bones, jawline and more linear features are softened by textured edges. An offset parting provides asymmetrical dimensions within the hairstyle. The colour of the eyes and hair are complementary. The head and hair shape sits comfortably on the contours of the model's shoulders.

Adopted techniques

The adopted techniques are mainly clubbing, graduation and texturising, particularly pointing and chipping in. The voluminous crown and top areas have been initially clubbed and blended into graduated layering at the nape and sides. Perimeter outlines have been softened using texturising techniques. Pointing has been used in the perimeter shape and chipping in provides lift in the internal style structure.

Apparent texture

The feel that radiates from the image is due to the contrast of the areas of smooth and chunky hair. The resultant effect is created by the application of product and cutting.

Movement and direction

The naturally straight hair has been given gentle movement throughout the shape.

Colour

Prisms semi-permanent chestnut and dark brown translucent colour gloss has been used.

Step-by-step guidance

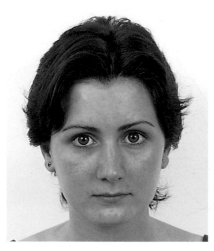

1 The client before the haircut.

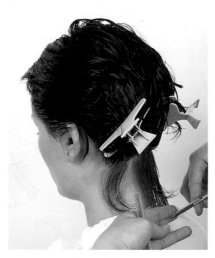

2 After shampooing and conditioning, section the nape hair horizontally. This determines the perimeter length.

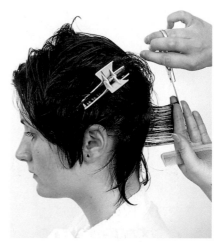

3 Take a section from the centre back. This provides the guideline of a reversed graduation, flaring out to the perimeter length.

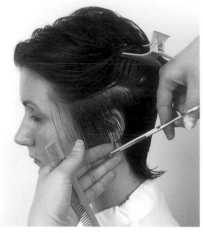

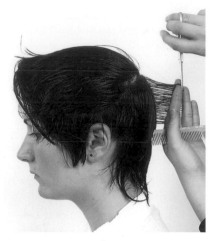

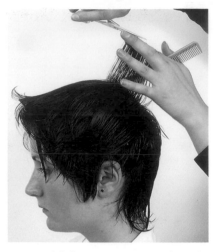

4 Take horizontal sections above the ear through to the temples and cut to provide a perimeter side baseline.

5 Continue taking sections up the back to beneath the crown, using graduation.

6 Hold the crown area directly out and club cut it.

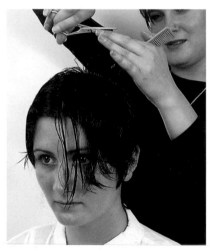

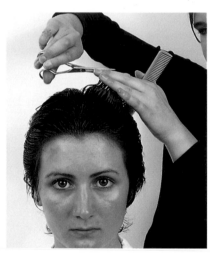

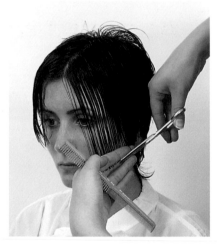

7 The crown section provides the guide.

8 Working towards the front, overextend the hair backwards on to the previously cut guide.

9 A natural parting denotes the boundary of the asymmetrical perimeter.

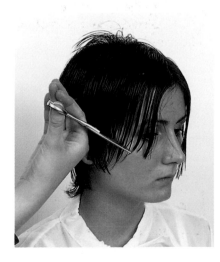

10 Shape the profile, moving from the long side to the shorter asymmetrical side.

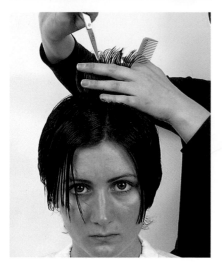

11 Serrate the club lines by pointing, providing lift and texture to the crown.

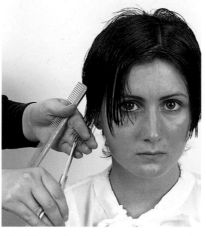

12 Soften the asymmetrical sides by pointing at the perimeter edges.

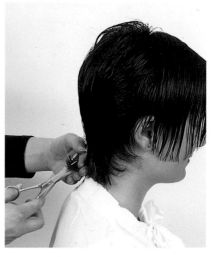

13 Continue pointing the nape hair.

MOULDING AND SHAPING

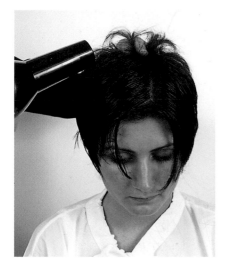

14 Apply volume and texture to the hairstyle by using rotary movements with fingers, hands and drier.

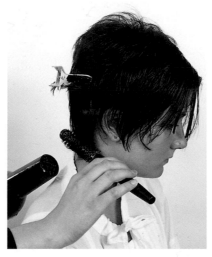

15 Use a small radial brush to create flickups at the back.

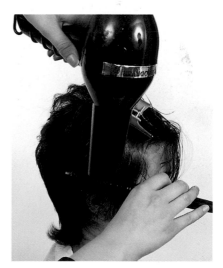

16 Dry the rest of the hairstyle using a small radial brush.

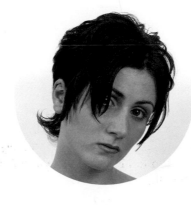

17 The final product effects have been achieved by using Fudge shaper on dry hair.

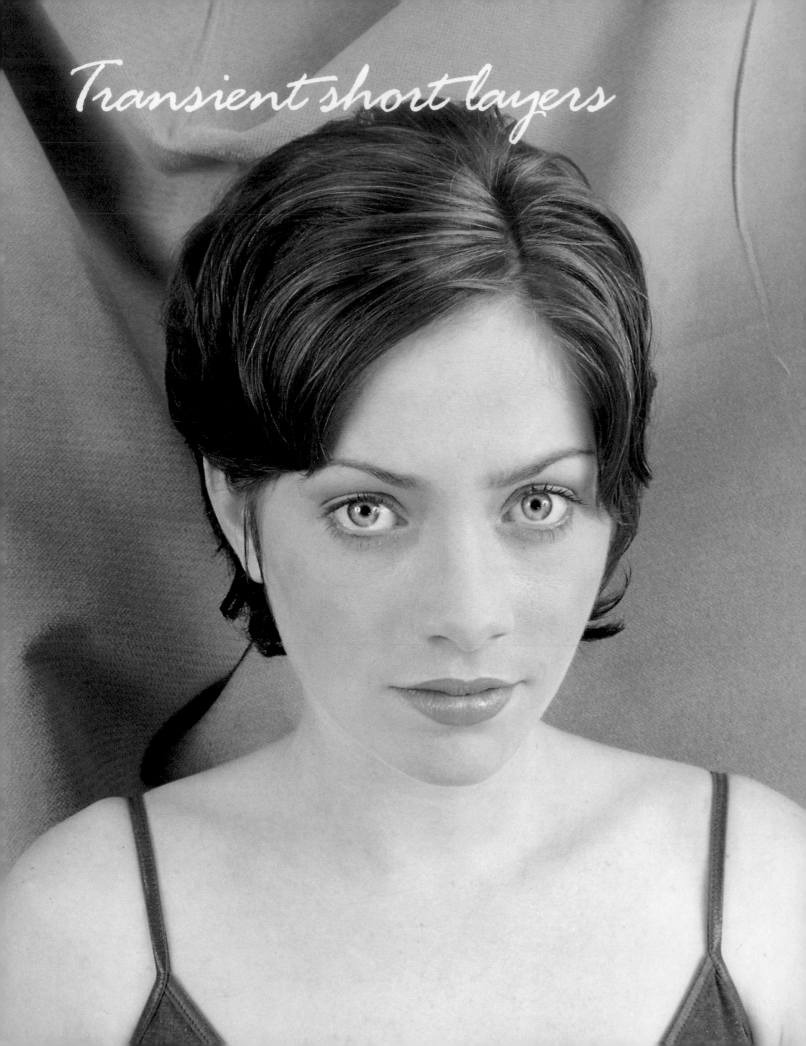

Transient short layers

Key building blocks

Shape and form

The fullness of the shape counterbalances the lines of the features of the head, particularly enhancing the focal point of the eyes.

Lines and angles

The lines of the chin and face merge with the movement, line and direction of the hair shape.

Colour depth and tone

The lightened tresses fully complement the line and direction of the hairstyle. The colour chosen for the low-lighting technique blends subtly with the darker hair and fair skin complexion. The range of cool tones blend well together.

Condition

The fluffiness of the hair is diminished by a final application of serum (Fudge licorice).

Step-by-step guidance

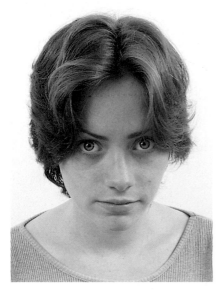

1 The client before the haircut.

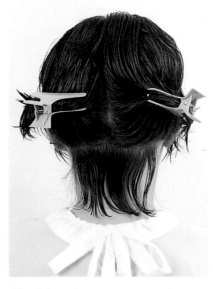

2 After shampooing and conditioning, section the nape hair horizontally, exposing the perimeter length to be cut.

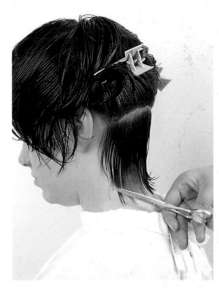

3 Cut it freehand to determine the length and shape of the perimeter.

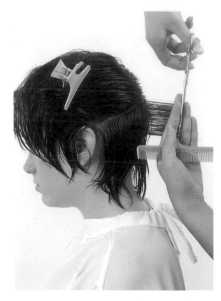 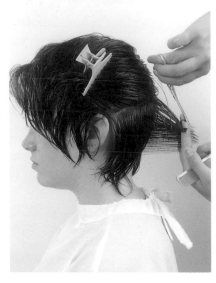 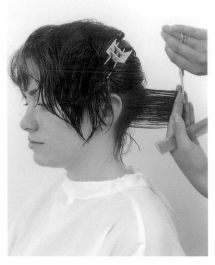

4 Take a section centrally at the back to provide a guide for the graduation.

5 Now reverse the angle, flaring it out to the length. This will help maintain bulk and weight.

6 Overextend the hair from behind the ears towards the centre to maintain weight behind the ears.

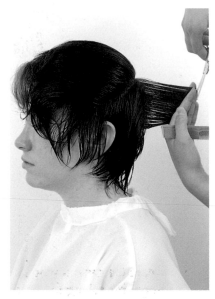 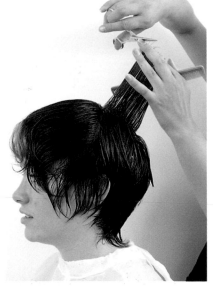 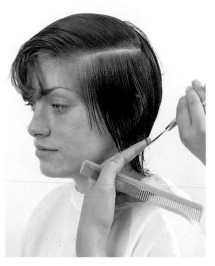

7 Take sections higher up the back, increasing the angle of graduation

8 Hold up the crown hair and club cut it. This provides a guide for the top layering.

9 Take a horizontal section at the side and blend the perimeter length into the back.

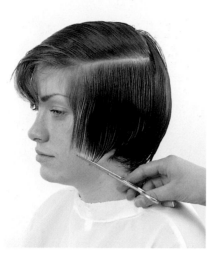

10 Complete the profile perimeter with freehand shaping around the face.

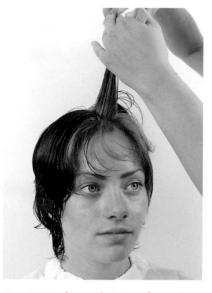

11 Make a division from the crown to the front, providing a guideline for the layering over the top.

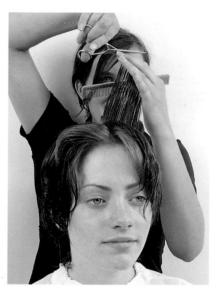

12 Blend the top length into the sides.

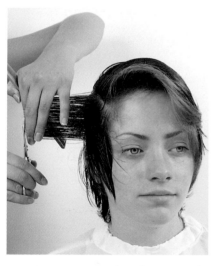

13 Continue the shaping of the sides with square layering.

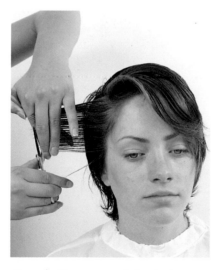

14 Overextend the hair back from the hairline to maintain the length around the face.

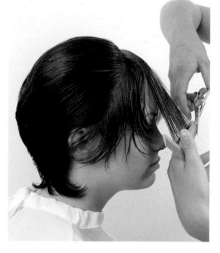

15 Retain the overall fringe length by pulling the hair forward and down, close to the face.

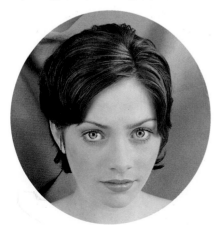

16 The finished look.

Short graduation

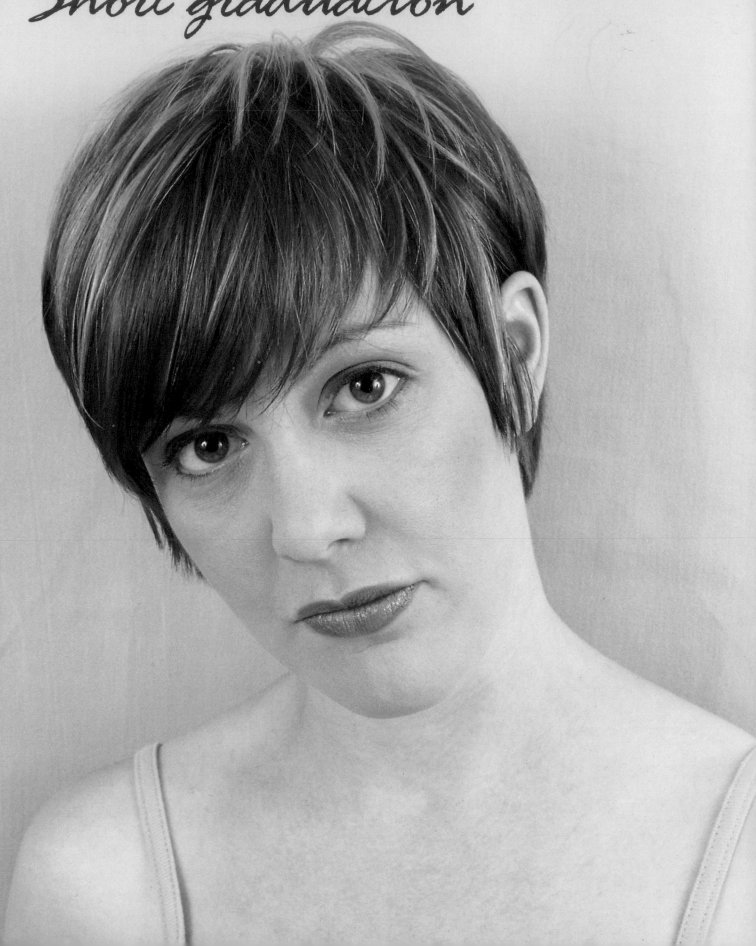

Key building blocks

Adopted techniques

The adopted techniques are mainly clubbing, graduation and texturising – particularly pointing. The voluminous crown and top areas have been initially clubbed and blended into graduated layering at the nape and sides. Pointing has also been used in the fringe and crown areas.

Apparent texture

The texture and feel of the hairstyle is greatly enhanced by the use of colour techniques.

Dimensions, distribution and abundance

The hair lifts at the crown and falls diagonally and asymmetrically forwards; the balance is maintained by creating extra lift and volume at the opposite side of the crown. The fringe and frontal area have ben left deliberately long to give a demure look.

Colour depth and tone

This particular effect has been created by layered colour techniques (see pages 92–3). The apparent contrast between light and dark hair, although subtle in appearance, has been achieved by using three not two colours. The effect is an illusion of light blonde on a vibrant red base. In this particular technique, light fronds of hair overfall sections of the third colour. This background enables dramatically contrasting colours to sit together in a pleasing way.

Step-by-step guidance

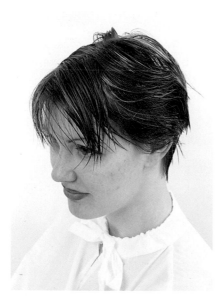 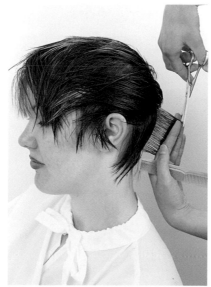 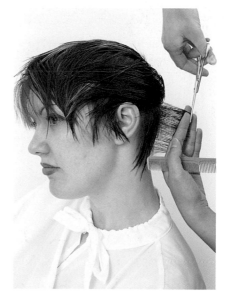

1 Shampoo and condition the client's hair.

2 Then section the nape hair horizontally. Take a vertical section at the centre of the back to provide a guideline for the graduation.

3 Continue the graduation through to the side, behind the ear.

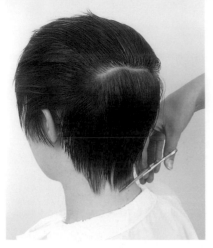

4 Complete the perimeter shape with freehand cutting.

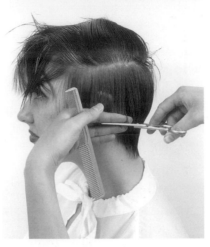

5 Take a horizontal section through to the side. Part of the graduated back hair provides a side perimeter guideline.

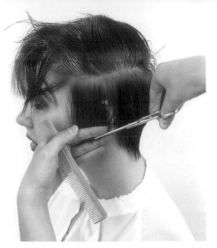

6 Continue the perimeter through to the front.

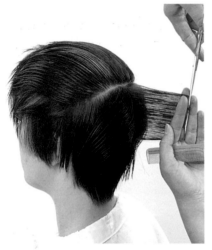

7 Section the hair higher at the back to continue the graduation.

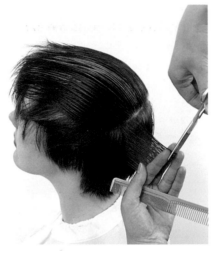

8 Continue this through to the side.

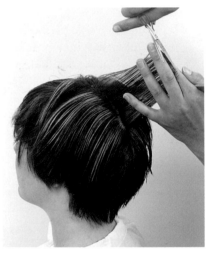

9 The previously graduated back hair now provides a guide to the overextended crown and top.

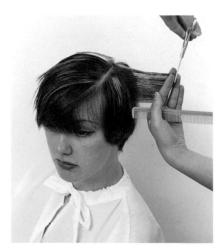

10 The previously graduated back sections also provide a guide for the top sides.

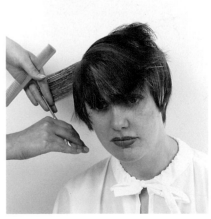

11 Continue this on the other side.

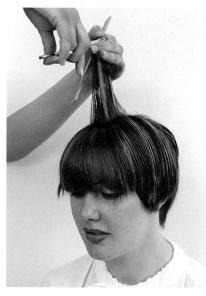

12 Maintain the top length by extending forwards from the pre-cut crown to the top front.

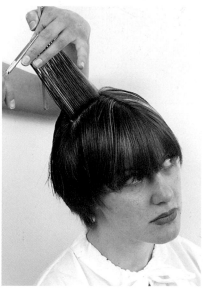

13 Take sections to the top.

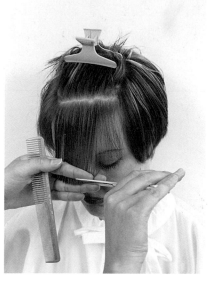

14 Determine the perimeter length for the fringe.

SPECIAL TECHNIQUES

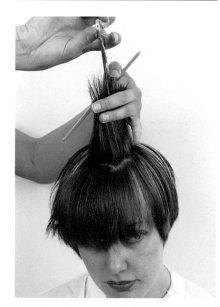

15 Texturise the crown area by pointing.

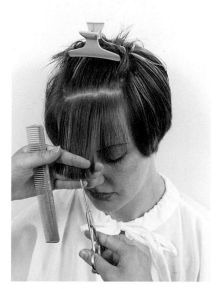

16 Texturise the fringe. Take a square base section and cut it by deep pointing.

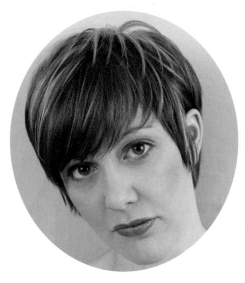

17 The finished look.

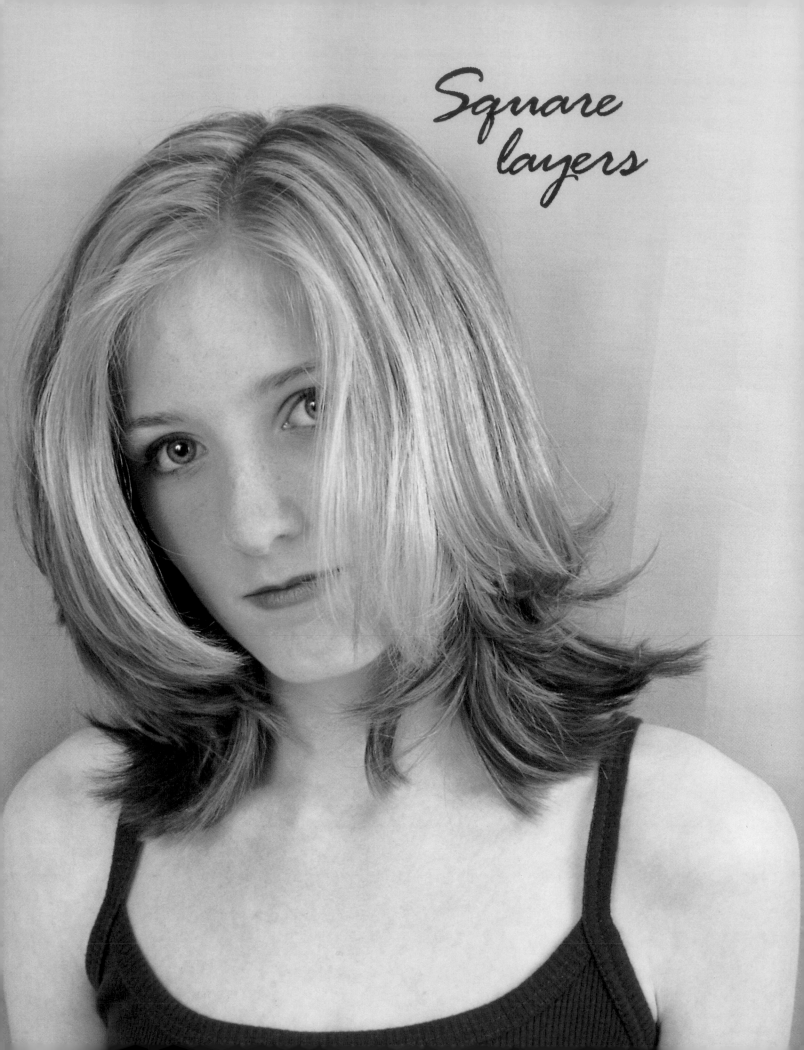

Square layers

Key building blocks

Shape and form

The overall hair frames the face and head. The length, with its softened edges, is allowed to fall naturally around the neck and shoulders. Contrast is drawn between sleek and smooth and soft and choppy areas.

Lines and angles

The direction in which the lines move puts the image into clear focus. The contour lines of the face, neck and shoulders are complemented by the style's movement.

Dimensions, distribution and abundance

An offset parting moves the weight of the hair to one side, softening the facial features. The body imparted by the cutting creates fullness.

Colour depth and tone

The softness of the effect is created by the contrast of light and dark. Only the surface hair in the parting area has been highlighted, simulating the effect that the sun has on hair. The rest of the soft layered hair remains strikingly dark. This is a good example of natural effects being produced artificially.

Step-by-step guidance

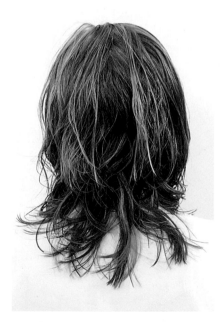

1 Shampoo and condition the client's hair.

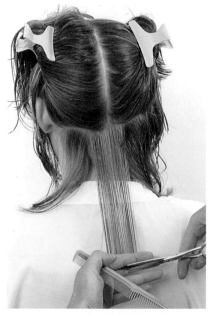

2 Then section the nape hair horizontally and cut a centrally perpendicular perimeter guide.

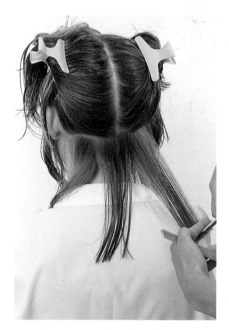

3 Continue the perimeter guide through to the sides.

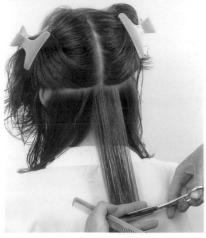

4 Take another section further up the back, providing a heavy perimeter shape.

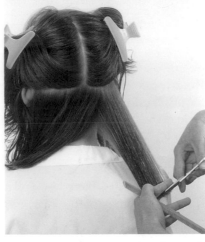

5 Again, continue this through to the sides.

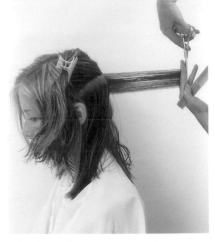

6 Start the square layering at this higher point.

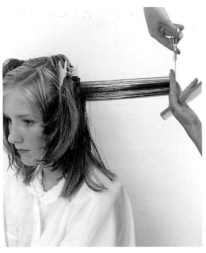

7 Continue cutting square layered sections around and above the ear.

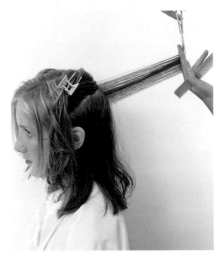

8 Continue up the back of the head.

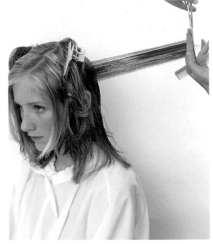

9 Continue through to the sides.

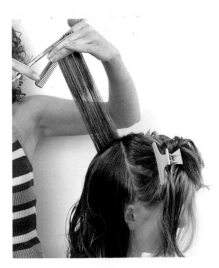

10 Cut square sections at the crown.

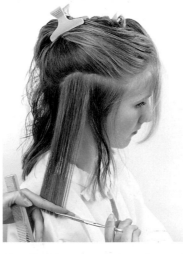

11 Use pre-cut hair from the back as a guide to perimeter length.

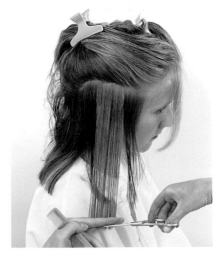

12 Continue this around the sides.

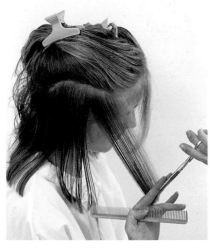

13 Extend the hair forwards to create a slight graduation.

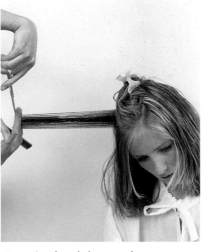

14 Blend the guide sections from the back into the sides.

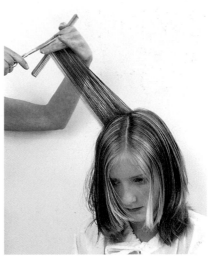

15 Continue the square layers up to the crown and parting.

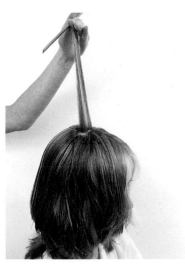

16 Cut the top overall length.

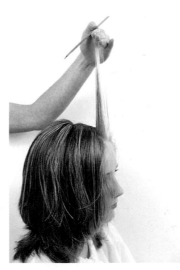

17 Continue sectioning through to the front perimeter.

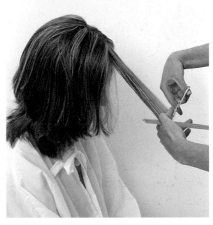

18 Shape the perimeter line around the front.

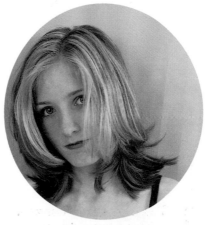

19 The finished look.

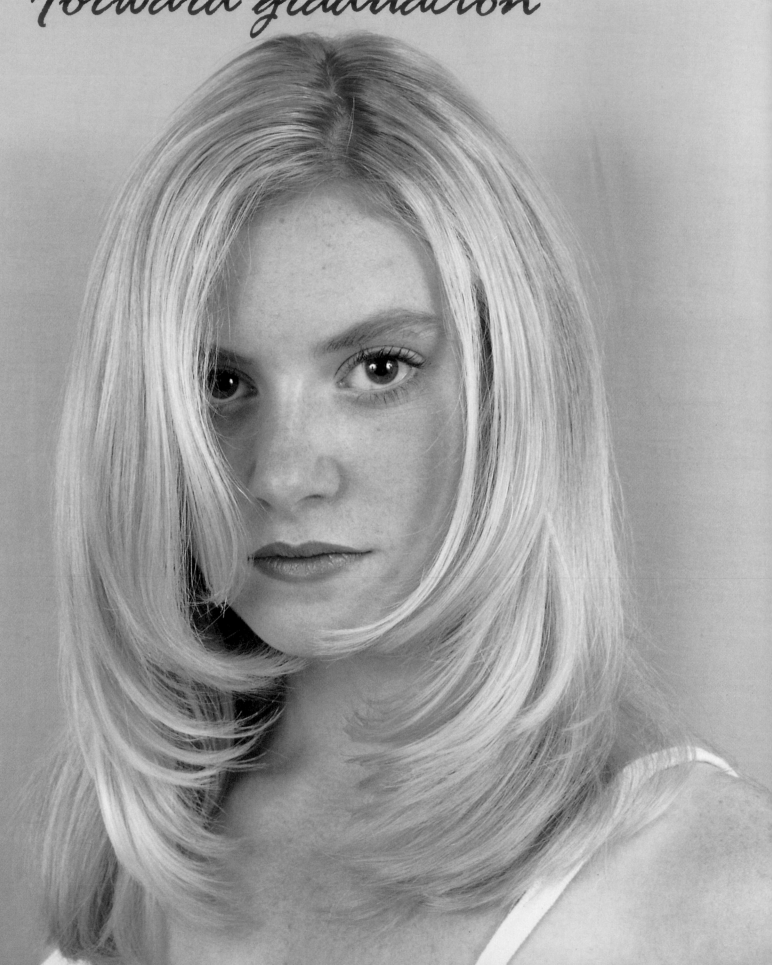

Forward graduation

Key building blocks

Lines and angles

The lines and angles of the hair shape emphasise the features of the face.

Movement and direction

The movement and direction of the style lines give vitality to the whole shape. Soft curving lines add extra appeal.

Colour depth and tone

The golden fronds are highlighted to emphasise line direction and movement.

Condition

The buoyant body and fullness is achieved by a velcro set: well-conditioned hair, carefully and smoothly wrapped, retains natural sheen and gloss.

Step-by-step guidance

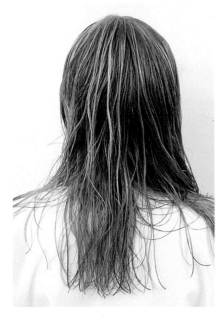

1 Shampoo and condition the client's hair.

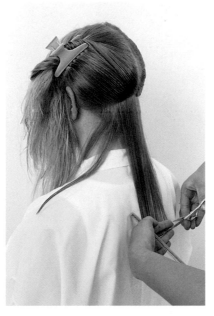

2 Then section the nape hair horizontally, exposing the perimeter length to be cut.

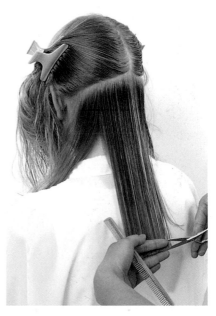

3 Take the next section horizontally behind the ears. Comb it down on to the previous guideline, and cut.

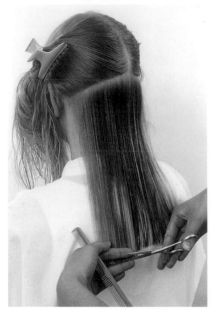

4 Extend this section behind the ears, completing the perimeter length.

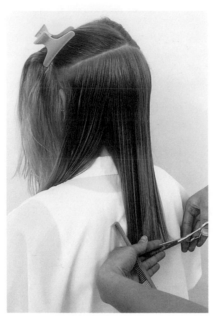

5 Shape further sections at the back of the head.

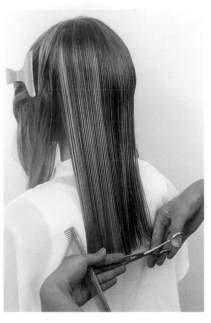

6 Continue this up to the top of the head.

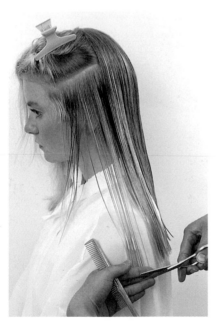

7 Take a horizontal section above the ear so that the side perimeter length may be determined.

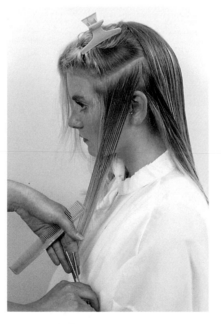

8 Hold the section forward to determine the perimeter graduation.

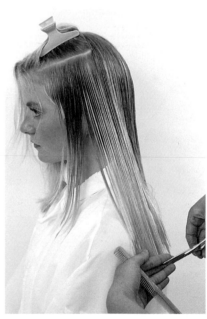

9 Take a horizontal section higher up the side.

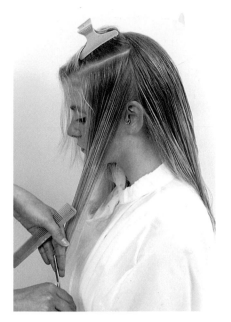

10 Then repeat step 8.

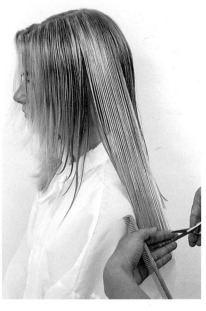

11 Continue up the side of the head until the parting is reached.

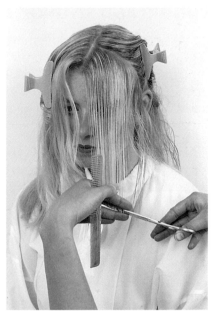

12 Trim the front perimeter graduation.

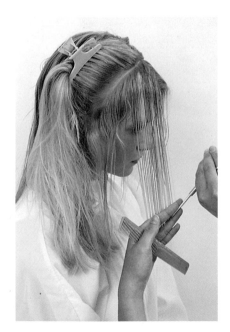

13 Repeat this on the other side of the head.

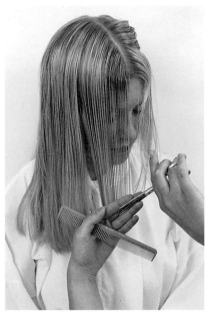

14 Continue until all the hair is cut.

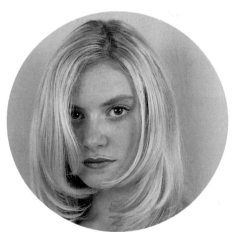

15 The finished look.

CUTTING AND STYLING

As you become more skilled in styling hair, you must remember that your work still rests on the accurate application of fundamental techniques, as well as on the more advanced ones you are now learning. Level 3 work is a continual process of building on experience. Fashion styling can now be attempted, but as always the following points must be considered:

- client communication
- determining baselines
- cutting tools and effects required
- methodical cutting
- cutting accuracy and checks
- client care
- health and safety.

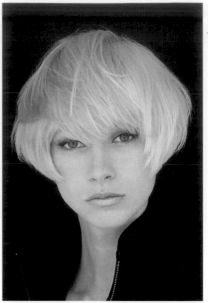

Communication with the client is an essential prerequisite to style cutting. In discussion with the client before any work takes place, you can determine what the client requires and thus what you need to do. You need to understand your client fully and negotiate with her throughout the service.

Be sure to listen to your client's requests. Many mistakes can be avoided at this stage if you achieve a clear understanding of what the client is asking for.

The hair cutting style that you choose with your client should take into account each of the following points:

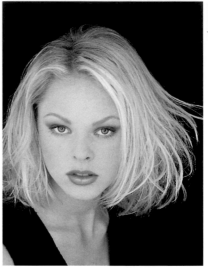

- the face and head shape
- face, head and body features
- what is appropriate to a given dress and occasion
- the quality and quantity of hair
- the client's age
- the hair's growth, position and proportion.

These factors are discussed in more detail in Chapters 1–3.

CUTTING BASELINES

It will be necessary to agree with your client the baselines to be cut.

A *baseline* is a cut section of hair which is used as a cutting guide for the following sections of hair. There may be one or more baselines cut: for example, a graduated nape baseline may be cut; another may be cut into the middle of the hair at the back of the head. Other baselines may be cut at the sides and the front of the head. The baselines will determine the perimeter of the hairstyle, or part of the style, and may take different shapes according to the effects required:

- *Symmetric* The baseline for evenly balanced hair shapes in which the hair is equally divided on both sides of the head. Examples are hairstyles with central partings or with the hair swept backwards or forwards.
- *Asymmetric* The baseline to be used where the hair is unevenly balanced, for example where there is a side parting

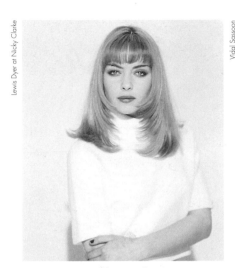

A symmetrical hairstyle

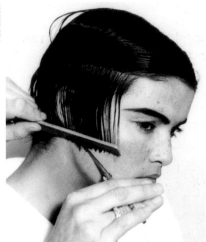

The side perimeter shape

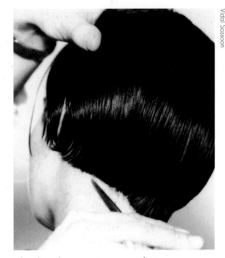

The back perimeter outline

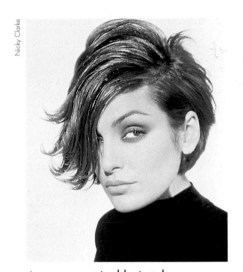

An asymmetrical hairstyle

and a larger volume of hair on one side of the head, or where the hair is swept off the face at one side with fullness of volume on the other.

- *Concave* The baseline may be cut curving inwards or downwards. The nape baseline, for example, may curve downwards.
- *Convex* The baseline may be cut curving upwards and outwards. The nape baseline, for instance, may be cut curving upwards.
- *Straight* The baseline may be cut straight across, for example where you wish to produce a hard, square effect.

CUTTING TOOLS

The choice of cutting tools is an individual one. It is important to select those that will enable you to achieve the specific effect that you want and to know what is required for the style or design that you are working on.

You must be able to control the cutting tool you select. It must be comfortable to hold and not too large to handle skilfully. The cutting edges must be sharp, or the hair will be torn and broken. Loose hair can be used to test the sharpness of scissor edges: if the blades cut cleanly, they are sharp enough; if the hair is bent or dragged during cutting, they are unacceptable.

Scissors

Scissors may be used to produce a variety of effects. Many scissors have serrated (sawlike) edges. If the serrations are small and fine, the scissors remove a small amount of hair with each cut; if they are large and coarse, the scissors remove a large amount of hair with each cut. *Thinning scissors* are designed to produce variation in the lengths in a section of hair: this gives tapered, thinned or texturised effects.

Cutting techniques reduce the length of some of the hairs in the section. The more hair removed, the more severe the effect of the cutting. The weight of the hair tends to straighten the hair, so the more you remove, especially towards the point ends of the hair section, the more the hair will tend to curl.

When you are tapering or thinning hair, remember not to remove hair lower (closer to the head) than the middle third of the hair section – unless you intend to produce a drastic effect. For most style cutting, tapering and texturising is kept to the point third of the hair section (that is, the third furthest from the head). When thinning, it is usually the middle of the hair section where most hair is removed.

Scissors are also used to produce clubbed effects – blunted ends of the hair sections. This technique retains the full weight of the hair at the ends. Non-serrated or finely serrated blades may be used to achieve clubbed effects. To ensure accuracy, take only small sections of hair each time you club cut, otherwise the cut line produced will be uneven. Although hair may be clubbed when it is either wet or dry, it is easier to control the hair when it is cut wet. Wet cutting is considered to be more hygienic, especially if it is done after cleaning the hair with shampoo.

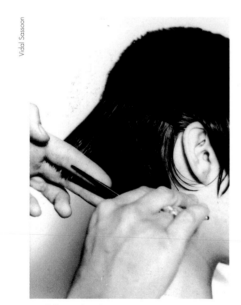

Holding the hair at the correct cutting angle for graduation

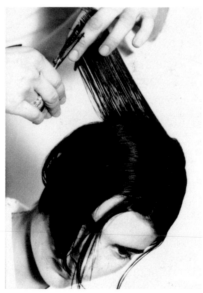

Clubbing – inner hair lengths

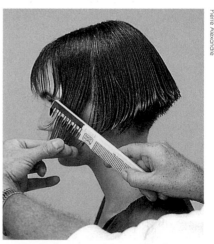

Cutting using a wide-toothed razor comb

Razors

Razors have traditionally been used to cut hair. They are mainly used to produce tapered, thinned and textured effects. The modern *hair shaper* is now replacing the traditional razor. This has exchangeable blades, which do away with the honing and stropping needed for open razors – the blade is always sharp and able to produce clean cuts. Although razors and hair shapers are mainly used to produce tapered and thinned effects, they can, with care, be used to produce clubbed effects too.

Razor cut

Trevor Sorbie

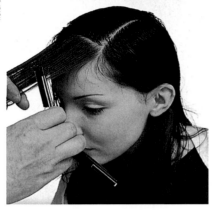

1 Start the cut at the front so the client can see the emerging shape. The horizontal angle of sectioning and the vertical angle of the cut are clearly visible.

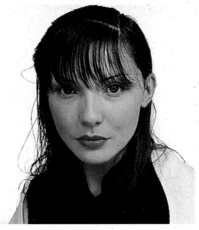

2 The effect produced is a very soft-edged outline.

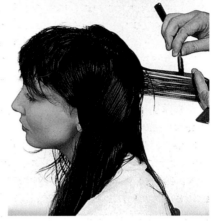

3 Graduate the hair section by holding it at a sharp angle to the head, fingers held at a 45° angle.

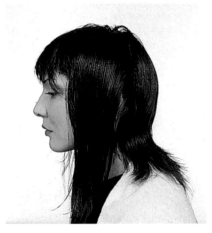

4 The effect produced is softly graduated ends.

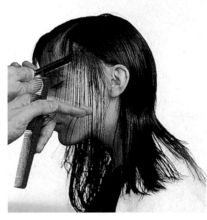

5 Shape the sides by holding the hair taut and close to the skin.

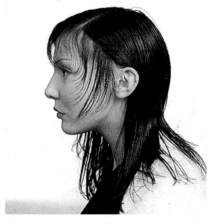

6 This is the effect produced by shaping.

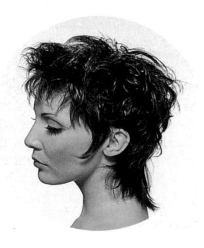

7 The finished effect can be produced by washing and leaving, by blow drying, by curling with small tongs for a more 'dressy' effect, or by waxing back for a 'sporty' effect.

Clippers

Clippers, which are either hand-operated or electric, are designed to produce clubbed hair effects. The closeness or shortness of the cut they produce is determined by the size of the cutting blades. With some clippers the blades are removable and designed to cut close to or further away from the head. Other clipper models have adjustable blades to determine the fineness of cutting.

A closely graduated effect in the nape may be produced using electric clippers or shapers. Alternatively, finely graduating the hair by cutting with scissors over a comb can be just as effective in achieving the style required.

SHAPING AND TEXTURISING

Removing bulk without affecting the length

To achieve this you should taper or thin the hair using scissors, thinning scissors or a razor. (Remember to use a razor only on wet hair.) Each of the texturising techniques – slicing, chipping, chopping, and so on – removes small amounts of hair bulk without reducing the overall hair length. These techniques should be used with thought and care to achieve the desired individual effects.

To remove bulk from long, thick hair, it is generally necessary to cut the hair at the middle third of the hair section. For more drastic thinning, the hair can be removed from nearer the roots. This can be achieved by point tapering, by razoring close to the scalp, or by using thinning scissors. On medium-length hair, removal of bulk can be achieved by cutting the hair about the middle section. To achieve bulk removal on short hair, you have to resort to root thinning.

Remember that razors can be used to remove hair from above or below sections.

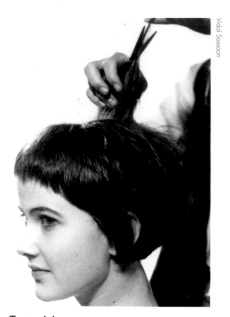

Texturising

Achieving lift and volume

To achieve lift and volume you need to reduce some of the hair lengths from each hair section. You can then use the shorter hairs as support for the longer hair. This applies particularly when you backdress the hair: the shorter hairs are more easily turned back to support the lengths. Thinning, tapering and texturising techniques can be used for these effects, on both short and medium-length hair.

Enhancing movement

For this you need to use tapered, thinned and texturised effects. Removing bulk hair, by tapering and thinning, encourages the remaining hair to curl more. This enables you to achieve tight, curly effects on long hair, and curl or waved effects on medium-length and short hair.

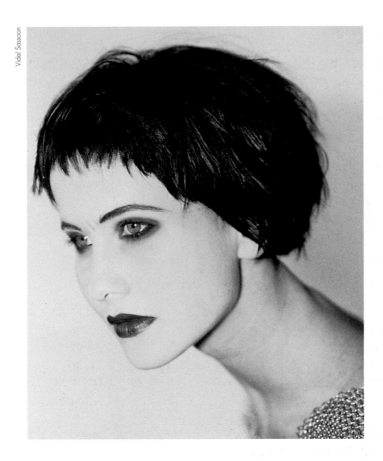

Vidal Sassoon

Producing non-uniform effects

Here you may use a variety or combination of texturising techniques: your choice will depend on the style effect that you want to produce. You must decide how much hair is to be removed, and how much you want to remain. Always remember that the head curves, from above to below and from side to side.

ACCURACY AND CHECKS

To achieve your agreed cut shape and style, you will need to carry out checks before, during and as you finish the cut. Without such care and continuity, unpredictable effects are likely to result.

Before the cut

- Communicate with your client and interpret her requests.
- Examine the hair – its type, length, quality, quantity and condition.
- Explain whether requests can or cannot be carried out.
- After further discussion, agree with the client exactly what is to be done.
- Try to show the hair length to be removed.
- Discuss the time that will be taken and the price that you will charge.

- Proceed only when all checks have been made and the client has agreed to your proposals.
- Ensure that you choose the correct tools and techniques – scissors for club cutting, razors for tapering and texturising, castle serrations for texturising, and so on.

During the cut

- To achieve precision cutting throughout, take care to check each angle at which the hair is taken and held from the head.
- Before you cut the hair section, be sure that it is at the angle you require.
- Your baselines and guideline cuts must be accurate as subsequent sections will be cut in relation to them. Think carefully before you make the first cut, and again before you follow on.
- When preparing baselines and guide sections, make sure that you attend to the features of your client's face and head. Use these as guides for accurate directions in the cut lines.
- Remember always that the first cuts you make often determine the finished shape of the style.

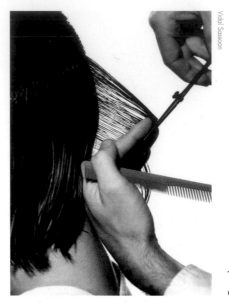

The holding and cutting angle

After the cut

- Check each of the sections of the side, nape, top and front for accuracy and finish.
- Carefully remove any straggly ends.
- Push and mould the hair as necessary to see the shape clearly.
- Satisfy yourself that you have achieved what was agreed.
- When all loose hair has been removed and the client is prepared and comfortable, continue to blow dry, set and finish the style.

Client care

You must take care at all times when you are working on your client. The client should be comfortable. She should never be apprehensive about what is being done: give your client your undivided attention.

Bear in mind the following points about client care:

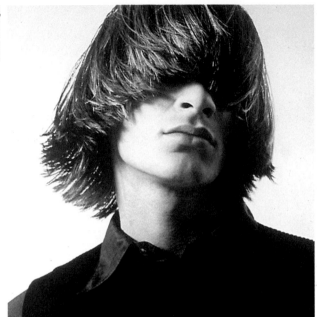

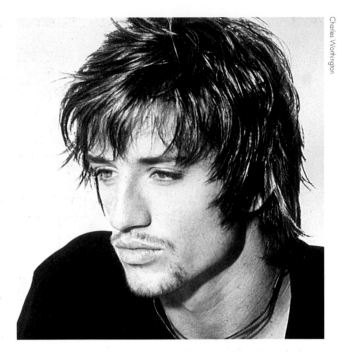

- Check the client's record card if she has attended the salon before. If this is a new client, make out a new record card.
- Protect the client adequately with cutting capes and gowns to prevent hair from spoiling clothes or causing irritation.
- All sharp-edged tools must be carefully used so that they never endanger the client.
- Talk to your client from time to time, explaining what is happening. Don't just ignore her and leave her to wonder.
- Aftercare is necessary if your client is to make the most of the cut style you have achieved. Suggest and show how the hair is best arranged and handled.
- Your client may wish to wash and condition the hair, or use hairsprays or hair cosmetics at home. Be prepared to offer professional guidance.
- Finally, give your client the opportunity to make the next appointment.

Health and safety

It is your responsibility to ensure your client's wellbeing and safety at all times. First and foremost, cross-infection must be avoided: this requires that you operate hygienically and carefully at all times. All tools and materials must be clean.

- Metal tools should be cleared of all hair and debris. They should be sterilised by being placed in an autoclave for the recommended time, or disinfected by cleaning with 70% alcohol wipes.
- Combs, brushes, plastic section clips and similar implements should be cleared of all hair, then washed and sterilised.

- Towels, gowns, wraps and other coverings must be freshly laundered. Only clean materials should be used on clients; they should then be discarded for washing or cleaning.
- It is important that you follow all the COSHH regulations and meet all other health and safety obligations, including the Health and Safety at Work Act 1974 and the Offices, Shops and Railways Act 1974. (See Chapter 14 for further details.)

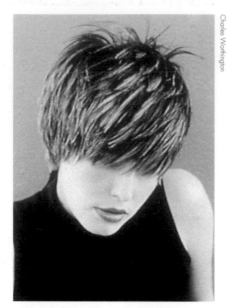

Charles Worthington

CHAPTER 5

Creative perming

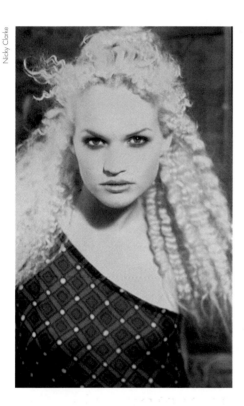

Nicky Clarke

INTRODUCTION

Modern technology provides the client with a number of options for the achievement of volume, movement and curl. This can be temporary, semi-permanent or permanent, depending on the product, chemistry and application involved.

The volume of scalp hair – its mass, bulk and dimension – is basically determined by the number of hairs present. This is an individual quality, which cannot be changed without resorting to added hair (postiche, hair extensions or hair transplants).

The movement of the hair is determined by the varying line and direction each hair takes: the growth patterns, or the amount of bend or curl present. Straight hair has little or no movement; wavy hair has a moderate amount of movement; curly or frizzy hair has the most movement. Fine straight hair lying close to and back from the forehead contributes little volume or bulk. A coarse textured head of hair which is frizzy will look as if it has more hair, but there may be the same number of follicle hairs on both heads. It is what is done with the hairs present that finally determines the volume effect of the hairstyle.

There are several ways in which volumising can be achieved, either temporarily or permanently. The temporary methods of volumising include chemical hair thickeners, bodifiers, and physical methods including thermostyling, setting, blow styling, hot brushes, tonging and heated rollers. The permanent methods of volumising are now mainly chemical: acid, alkaline, cold, tepid and hot methods.

In this chapter we provide step-by-step guidance to creative perming, as well as relevant background information. The building blocks you need to consider include:

Shape and form

Lines and angles

Adopted techniques

Apparent texture

Movement and direction

Dimensions, distribution and abundance

Twist and roll using hair formers

Key building blocks

Shape and form

The symmetrical balance is obtained by dividing the hair centrally. The length is maintained by using large formers – foam-covered rollers – which produce a loose, open curl.

Adopted techniques

The fine hair is point wound, both twisting and rolling along the hair section.

Apparent texture

The apparent texture is achieved by alternating the use of different hair curl former sizes.

Step-by-step guidance

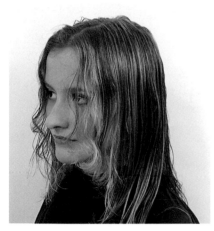

1 After shampooing and towel drying, divide the hair centrally.

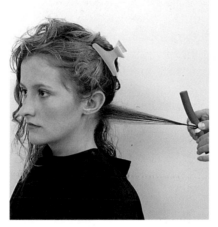

2 Take the first small rectangular section cleanly out from the nape and secure the point ends to the former.

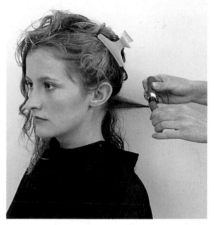

3 Wind the hair for one complete turn and then twist it through half a turn until the nape is reached.

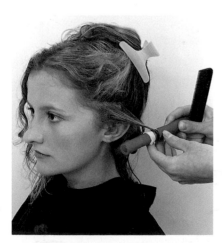

4 Position the former, then continue rolling and twisting from one side of the nape to the other.

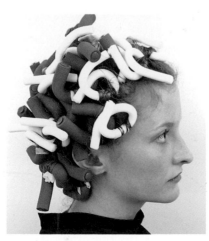

5 The completed wound head.

THE BACKGROUND TO PERMING

Permanently curling hair goes back to the beginning of civilisation. Early Egyptians wound hair around sticks, coated it with clay, and baked it in the sun. The old wigmakers and perruquiers found that wrapping hair on sticks and boiling it produced a permanent curl.

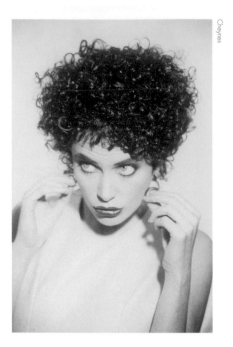

Hot perming systems

Early this century, a perming system was introduced which consisted of winding hair in spirals from roots to points around sticks, bigoudies or curlers, secured by tying the ends with string. Borax paste was coated on to the wound hair. Muslin, paper or flannel was used to cover and protect it. Heat was then applied to each wound curler and allowed to cool. Tongs and crimping irons were originally used to apply the heat. These were later replaced by electric heaters.

Such systems were used in a variety of forms up to the end of the 1940s. The first systems had the disadvantage of excessive heat, used over long periods. Dry hair and burnt scalps also resulted. Early electric machines produced shock and discomfort. Systems were later introduced which used lower alkaline lotions, lower temperatures, better curlers, protective water curlers and safer electric machines.

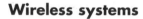

Wireless systems

The newer systems ended the need for clients to be attached by wires to a machine. They required the hair to be wound from points to roots, croquignole fashion. Kinder reagents were used, and the heat was supplied by heaters detached from a machine. Specially designed clamps which fitted over the wound curler were heated up instead.

Tepid perming

This was introduced at about the same time as wireless and machineless systems, but it did not rely on a machine for its heated clamps. It used croquignole winding and the application of a reagent which was like a cold, weak perm lotion. The wound curlers were covered with sachets of this lotion, which were activated by immersing them in water. The sachets contained calcium oxide, and the heat generated activated the reagents used on the hair.

Tepid perming was known as the first 'exothermic' system. Although it did not achieve great acclaim initially, it gradually grew in popularity. The advantages of the tepid system were the lower alkaline reagents used, the lower heat, the better condition of the hair afterwards, and the general improvement in client comfort and safety.

Rita Rusk

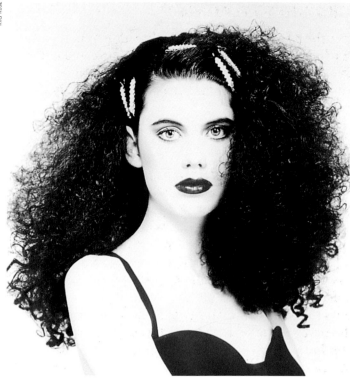

The cold perming or waving system (CPW)

This was introduced on a large scale in about 1940. It consisted of a reagent applied to wound curlers, with less winding tension, and it required another oxidising neutralising lotion to be applied to stop its action when sufficient wave formation was achieved. It was initially harsh and rough, and produced many unwanted frizzed heads of hair.

Today's cold perms are vastly superior, and the hair is left in much better condition, with natural looking effects.

Semi-permanent or demi-wave systems

Neville Daniel

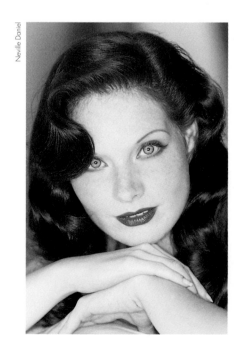

These have been introduced in different forms over the years. They produce curl or wave which gradually fades over six to eight weeks. They have proved popular, because they create gentle effects and enough body to hold modern styles. They rely on the use of large curlers and cold-waving type lotions, activated by the heat from the head, hood dryer, or rollerball, accelerator, climazone and infra-red dryers.

Alkaline and acid perms

The systems we currently use to perm hair rely on alkaline- or acid-based activating lotions, applied to a variety of curler shapes and sizes. They are activated by a range of more gentle temperatures than those used in the past. Normalising solutions are used to stop the processing and return the hair to its normal state.

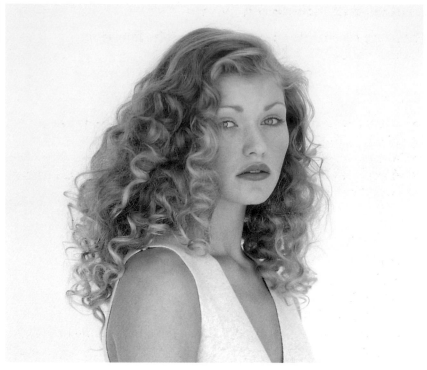

Alkaline

- Effective on strong, coarse, resistant hair which is difficult to wave.
- Alkaline lotion, up to pH 9, is suitable for different hair textures.
- The lotion swells the hair, lifts the cuticle and penetrates to the cortex.
- Less winding tension is required.
- Croquignole and spiral winds can be used.
- The test curl forms a stronger, sharper shape.
- The hair must be normalised or neutralised.
- The higher the pH and the stronger the lotions, the more potential there is for damage.
- No additional heat is required.

Acid

- Suitable for fine, delicate, porous and previously chemically processed hair.
- Shrinks hair and smoothes cuticle.
- Some require additional heat to be applied: climazone, rollerball, accelerator or infra-red dryer.
- Make sure that the reagents are activated by mixing the solutions correctly: check with the manufacturer's instructions.
- The test curl forms a softer, looser shape – a crisp, snappy test curl could result in overprocessing.
- Needs a longer processing time than alkaline perms.
- Pre-damp or post-damp – more often post-damp.

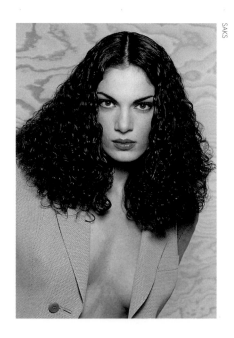

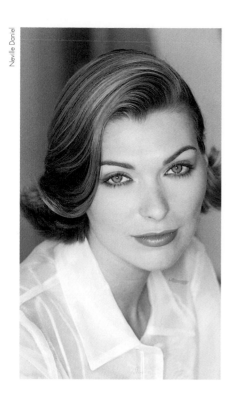

Neville Daniel

Neutral and techniwave perms

These are recent introductions and have the following characteristics.

Neutral

- Special wavers ensure the tension in the hair is correct.
- Reduces the amount of ammonia that is present.
- Minimises the swelling of the hair.
- A near neutral pH combines the gentle benefits of acid perms with the long-lasting effects of alkaline perms.

Techniwave

- Permanent style support.
- Maintains a lasting affinity to the hair fibre.
- Neutraliser contents contribute to good condition, management and lasting results.
- Special wavers make sure that the tension in the hair is correct.

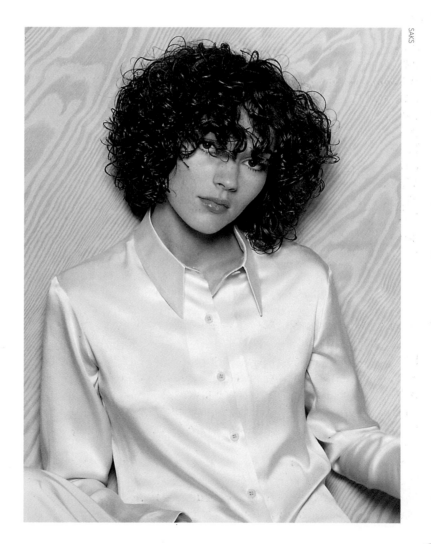

SAKS

Other types of perm which give volume support

- *Root perms* Perming the lower root ends of the hair. The hair is wound at the root ends only; the point ends are left out and not processed. This allows the hair to produce fullness and volume. Reperming must be kept strictly to the regrown root ends.
- *Body perms* The root and middle hair lengths can be processed to give added body to the hair.
- *Pin perms, roller perms, semi- or demi-perms* These involve the application of a weaker form of perm lotion, which lasts for six to eight weeks. Reprocessing can take place through the hair lengths after this time has elapsed. These are not intended to be permanent, but to produce body fullness.

PERMING TECHNIQUES

Spiral curls

The spiral curl is both a traditional and a current style effect. It may be produced by temporary and permanent techniques.

The temporary spiral curl is produced by setting the hair on to curlers, rods, sticks, or pliable or bendable curl formers. Setting aids such as mousse, gel or lotion can be used to extend the life of the spiral curl thus made.

Permanent spiral curls are produced by the application of chemical permanent waving techniques. As with all style effects, client consultation should ensure that what is agreed takes account of the relevant factors.

Selecting the size and position of the curls

The spiral curl is dependent on the length of the client's hair. If the hair is less than 10 cm long it will be difficult, and perhaps impossible, to form spiral shapes of any size. Hair longer than 10 cm will permit reasonable spiral formations: longer hair will enable fuller, thicker and longer curls to be shaped.

The position that these spiral curls take and the overall effect that they produce must be discussed with your clients: you must ensure that they understand exactly what is being done. They should also know before they leave the salon how to maintain the perm.

Spiral curls may be formed all over the head – length permitting – or they may be formed and positioned to form a cascade in the nape. Alternatively, bunches of spiral curls may be positioned asymmetrically. The degree of the spiral curl shape and the effect finally produced is for you and your client to determine jointly at the outset.

Tools

The tools required for producing permanent spiral curls – in addition to those required for general cold perming – will be whatever type of curler, rod or curl former you choose to use. Formers are available in a variety of shapes and sizes: some are screw-shaped; some are square; others are long or flat.

Your choice of curl former is determined by the effects that you wish to create. Think about this carefully before attempting the perm.

Starting the wind

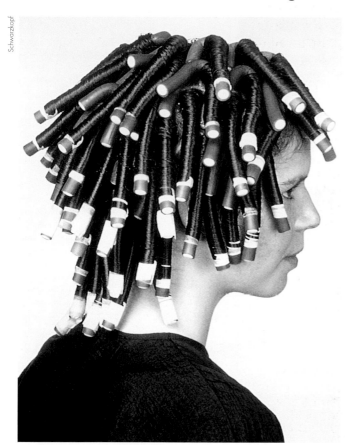

A completed spiral wind

The spiral wind can be started at the root end of the hair, or from the hair points. If you use a curl former that is of the same thickness overall, the curl you produce will be even throughout. If you use a former that tapers or is concave, the results will be uneven.

For the resultant curl to be even, springy and smooth, your winding must be firm, without undue tension, wrapped cleanly over the former and secured without indenting or marking the wound hair.

If you apply uneven tension to your winding, the spiral formation will be inconsistent – the loops and turns will not follow on and there may be gaps in the shape.

Securing the wind

When you secure the hair formers, be careful not to cut into the wound hair – breakage could result if you did. Follow the recommendations of the makers of the curl former that you are using. You must also ensure that the formers are secured firmly: if they are loose, the hair may drop or unwind.

Monitoring the perm process

Once you have completed your winding and secured the formers, you must monitor the perm process. If the perm lotion is applied to the hair before winding – a technique called *pre-damping* – the winding must be carried out without delay. Alternatively, the lotion can be applied after the winding is complete – *post-damping*. Perm processing is always timed from the moment the lotion is applied.

You will need to check the development of the perm process. You can achieve this by taking a test curl. By gently unwinding the hair part-way you can check the development of the 'S' shape. If the shape is loose then further development may be required. If the shape is well formed, begin normalising straightaway: the perm is said to have 'taken'.

As well as monitoring the timing carefully, you must:

- ensure your client's comfort
- keep excess lotion off the skin
- remove damp cottonwool (used to protect the skin) when it has absorbed the lotion, or scalp 'burns' will occur
- continually reassure the client so that she never feels she has been forgotten
- use a timer which makes an audible noise when the time has elapsed.

Normalising

When the perm has taken, you must stop the perming process quickly. This is an important stage. If you are supervising a junior hairdresser, be sure to doublecheck with her that she is monitoring whether the perm has taken and is ready to normalise the hair.

Normalising should include the following stages:

1 Rinse the wound hair thoroughly with warm water to remove the perm lotion. Make sure the water is not too hot or there may be a sudden tightening of the perm.
2 Blot the curlers or formers to remove surplus water, using tissues or towels. (If this is not done the normaliser may become diluted and the perm is likely to drop.) When monitoring others, ensure that this has been done thoroughly.
3 Apply the normaliser as recommended by the manufacturer. Care must be taken that it covers *all* of the wound hair. Ensure that the curlers in the nape and around the ears are not missed.
4 When you have completed the normaliser application, start the timing. The time the normaliser should remain on the hair varies with the type and make of the perm used: make sure that you know the recommended time for the normaliser you are using.
5 When the first application of the normaliser has been on the hair for its allotted time, the curlers may be removed. This must be done with care as the hair may still be soft. Harsh handling could weaken the perm.
6 You may now apply the second stage of

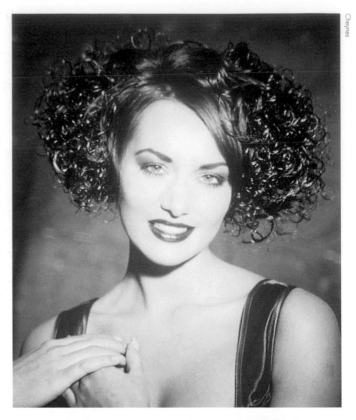

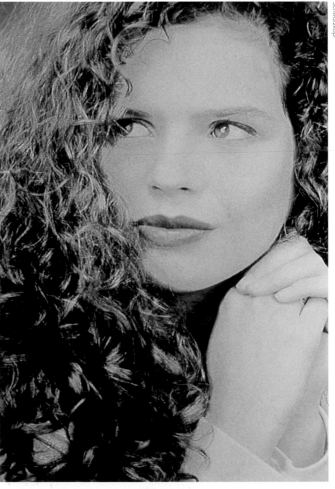

normalising. This too must be carefully timed. Again, check that the normaliser has covered all the hair.

7 Now rinse the hair well to remove all traces of normaliser. At this stage the hair may be conditioned and made ready for setting for blow styling.

Problems

Below are some problems that you may meet when producing permanent spiral curls:

- *The root end is straight* You can avoid this by securing the former firmly at the root end of the hair. The helical loops of hair will be too loose if they are not firmly wound and in close contact with the former.
- *Hair 'kicks' out* Ensure that the hair is not twisted when you form the spiral curl. After each turn, the hair should be repositioned. If you allow the hair to twist, an irregular spiral will be formed: this could cause the hair to stick out from the head. It is difficult to remedy this afterwards.
- *The spiral curl is too loose* Provided that the hair condition permits it, the hair may be reprocessed. You must take special care if you do this as the hair will be far more receptive to the perm lotion and could easily become overprocessed.

Perming hair of different lengths

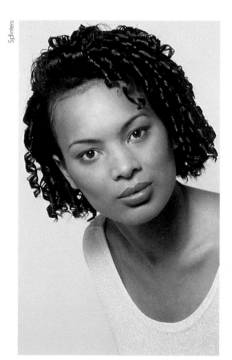

Splinters

Short lengths of hair (less than 10 cm) are not suitable for permanent spiral curls because it is impossible to form the helical shape on the curl former.

Medium hair lengths (10–15 cm) do allow spiral formations. These are likely to be short and narrow.

Longer lengths of hair (15 cm and longer) are the most suitable. Here there is sufficient hair to produce a variety of full, long, springy shapes. Greater lengths allow the hair to be placed on to the former more easily, and a wider variety of curl formers may be used.

Direction and degree of movement

The direction of perm movement is determined by the angle that you wind and position the curlers or rods. If a forward direction of the fringe area is required, the wound curlers must be positioned accordingly.

The degree of perm movement is the 'tightness' or 'looseness' of the wave or curl. This is determined by:

- the size of curlers, rods or formers used
- the time for which the hair is processed
- the amount of tension used
- the hair texture and its condition
- the perm lotion strength
- the type of winding used.

Small curlers produce small wave shapes; large curlers produce large wave shapes. The longer the perm process, the tighter the curl or wave shape – but remember that if left too long the hair could become overprocessed, causing poor condition, loss of elasticity and weakening of the hair. Stretching or tensioning the hair will produce tighter results; winding without tension produces looser results.

Choice of perm lotion

The texture and condition of the hair determines the degree to which the perm lotion used is absorbed. Fine hair in poor condition with a torn cuticle is likely to absorb perm lotion quickly. Coarser hair with a smooth cuticle is likely to take much longer to process: it is more resistant to the perm lotion.

Manufacturers produce perm lotions of varying strengths. Some are designed for fine hair; others for medium or coarse hair. Others still are designed for use on chemically processed hair, such as hair that has been bleached or coloured.

Your choice of permanent waving lotion is therefore important. First determine what state the hair is in. If you decide that the hair is in good condition and that it is of medium texture, you may choose the perm lotion for normal hair. If you find that the hair is fine and has a lifted cuticle, use a lotion recommended for fine hair or hair in poor condition. Bear this in mind also as you determine the curler size, the tension of the wind and the processing time. If the hair is thicker or coarser and has a smooth cuticle, there may be some resistance to the lotion and the hair will take longer to process. Choose the manufacturer's lotion for coarse hair.

The surest way to determine the end result is by taking test curls. Either cut a piece from the hair to be permed or section a small area at the back of the head. Determine the hair texture, condition, type of perm, processing time, curler size, type of winding, and so on; then process the test curls. Make a note of what is being done so that the curl or wave produced can then be repeated for the whole head of hair.

When making test curls, be sure to select an area where the hair is not unduly different from that on the rest of the head. Note, however, that there may be specific areas of weakened hair that you may wish to test separately. If you make a test curl with hair cut from the head, make allowance for the lack of body heat – the processing time for the whole head may not be the same as that for the test curl.

Perming problems and solutions

	Possible cause	Immediate action	Future action
Hair/scalp damage			
Breakage	Too much tension or bands on curlers too tight. Hair overprocessed – chemicals far too strong	Apply restructurant or deep-action conditioner to remainder of hair	Use less tension. Review choice of lotion, timing, etc.
Pull burn	Perm lotion allowed to enter follicle. Tension on hair excessive	Apply soothing moisturiser to affected area. If condition serious, refer to doctor	Use less tension. Take smaller meshes
Sore hairline, skin irritation	Chemicals allowed to come into contact with skin. Poor scalp ventilation	Consult regarding allergies, then apply soothing moisturiser to affected area. If condition serious, refer to doctor	Curlers to rest on hair, not skin. Keep lotion away from scalp. Renew cottonwool after damping
Straight frizz	Lotion too strong for hair. Excessive winding tension. Hair overprocessed	Cut ends to reduce frizz. Apply restructurant or penetrating conditioner	Ensure appropriate lotion is used in future. Wind with less tension. Time carefully
Perm result/effect			
Too curly	Curlers too small. Lotion too strong	If hair condition allows, reduce curl amount by relaxing	Ensure appropriate curlers and lotion are used
No result	Lotion too weak or not enough used. Curlers too large. Poor neutralising. Hair underprocessed	If hair condition allows, reperm hair with suitable lotion	Use appropriate lotion and rods. Process perm and neutraliser in line with manufacturer's instructions
Fish-hooks	Hair points not wrapped properly. No end papers	Remove ends by cutting	Check points of hair are wrapped correctly. Use end papers
Perm weakens	Poor neutralising. Hair stretched excessively while drying	If hair condition allows, reperm hair	Check method and timing of neutraliser. Do not over-stretch while drying hair
Good result when wet, poor when dry	Hair stretched while drying. Ineffective neutralising. Overprocessed	If hair condition good, reperm. Apply conditioning agents to moisturise hair	Check method and timing of neutraliser and perm lotion. Avoid stretching while drying
Uneven curl	Uneven winding technique. Uneven tension. Uneven lotion application. Ineffective neutralising.	If hair condition allows, reperm affected area	Check wound curlers before applying perm lotion or neutraliser
Straight pieces	Lotion not applied evenly. Rods too large	If hair condition allows, reperm affected area	Ensure even lotion application
Colour			
Hair discoloured	Metal tools or equipment allowed to contact hair. Metallic dye present in hair	Tone hair to correct shade. Apply semi-permanent	Carry out incompatibility test. Use plastic and rubber equipment only for perming

Perming techniques: quick reference guide

Perm technique	Final effect	Ideal length	Lotion type	Equipment
Root	Lift and body at root area only	Layered hair or graduated hair, 100–150 mm long	Acid or alkaline; often used as a thick cream or paste	Conventional rods, often used with non-porous end papers
Pincurl	Lift and body with soft movement at ends	Layered hair of a uniform length, 50–75 mm long	Acid or alkaline; often used as a thick cream or paste	Aluminium or plastic pin clips
Directional*	Lift and body with definite forced movement at ends	Layered or graduated hair, 100–150 mm long	Acid or alkaline	Conventional or oval-type rods
Weaving	Textured soft and stronger movement within the style	Layered or graduated hair, over 75 mm long	Acid or alkaline	Conventional or oval-type rods
Piggyback (double wind)	Textured curl with varying curl diameters	Layered or graduated hair, over 75 mm long	Acid or alkaline	Conventional or oval-type rods
Stack	Very little root movement with strong end curl	Graduated 150 mm at crown down to 50 mm at nape	Acid or alkaline	Conventional rods
Zigzag	Strong geometric, angular movement	One length or long, layered hair: 250 mm minimum length	Alkaline	Perming mats or chopsticks
Spiral	Cascades of curls with a firm uniform curl diameter	One length or long, layered hair: 250 mm minimum length	Alkaline	Spiral rods and foam-covered flexible wavers

*Used also to determine 'root' direction (e.g. around side hairline to direct hair away or upwards from face).

Winding and the
finished effects

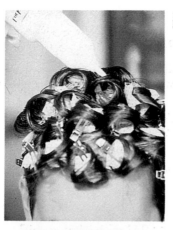

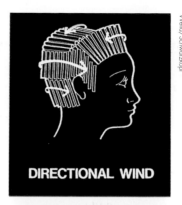

DIRECTIONAL WIND

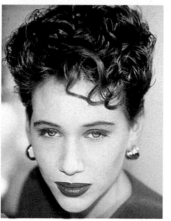

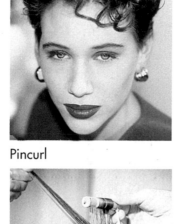

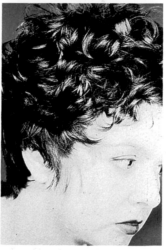

Pincurl

Directional wind

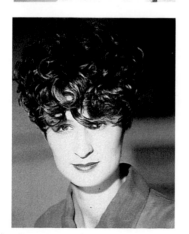

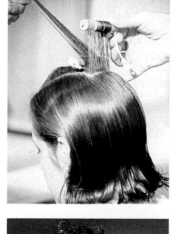

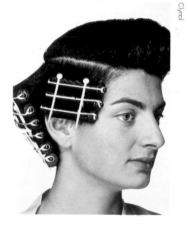

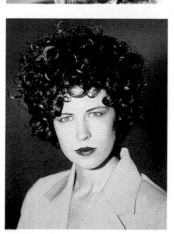

Weave wind

Double wind

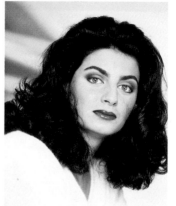

Stack wind

Alternative perming techniques

The curl shape and structure achieved using conventional perm rods with traditional (croquignole) winding techniques will usually be uniform in its appearance. The only exception is directional winding, which is possible with conventional rods.

For special perming techniques you need to use alternative perming systems. Here are some examples.

Spiral rods

1 Take a small rectangular section of hair.
2 Place a rod hook over the hair and slide it towards the scalp.
3 Wind hair around the rod.
4 Secure the ends with a spiral clip.
5 Repeat steps 1–4 to complete the entire head.

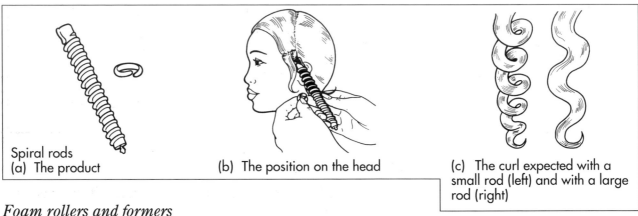

Spiral rods
(a) The product

(b) The position on the head

(c) The curl expected with a small rod (left) and with a large rod (right)

Foam rollers and formers

1 Take a small rectangular section of hair.
2 Secure the hair points in an end paper.
3 Wind the hair around the roller.
4 Secure the roller by bending it over.
5 Repeat steps 1–4 to complete the entire head.

Clynol

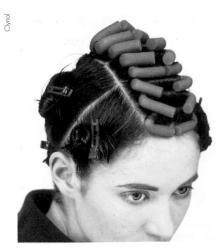

Formers
(a) The formers being wound on

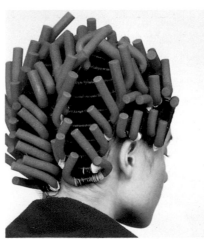

(b) Winding complete

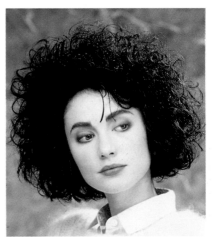

(c) The finished effect

Crimpers

1 Take a conventional winding hair section, no wider than the crimpers.
2 Place the open crimper, with its spikes facing upwards, under the hair section.
3 Place an end paper on the ends of the hair section and close the crimper.
4 Depending on the hair length, continue with extra crimpers.
5 Repeat steps 1–4 to complete the entire head.

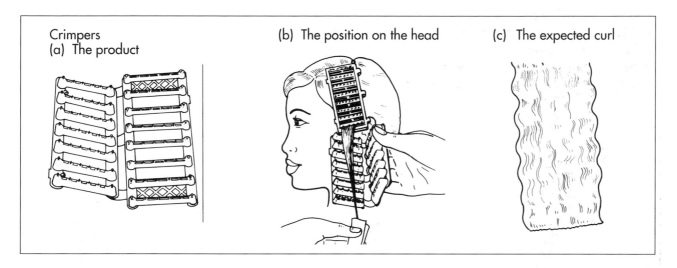

Crimpers
(a) The product

(b) The position on the head

(c) The expected curl

Chopsticks

1 Take a small square section of hair and protect it with one or more end papers.
2 Place the hair section through the loop and hold it securely.
3 Separate the chopstick 'legs' and wind the hair in a figure of eight.
4 Secure the end paper on to the chopsticks using a rubber band.
5 Repeat steps 1–4 to complete the entire head.

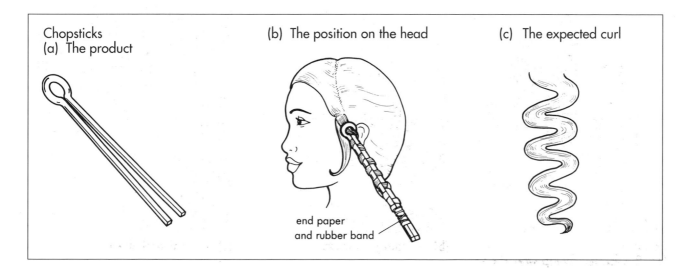

Chopsticks
(a) The product

(b) The position on the head

(c) The expected curl

end paper
and rubber band

U-stick rods

1 Take a small square section of hair and pull it through the middle of the U-stick.
2 Wind the hair in a figure-of-eight movement around the U-stick.
3 Protect the ends with one or more end papers.
4 Secure the end papers on the U-stick with a rubber band.
5 Repeat steps 1–4 to complete the entire head.

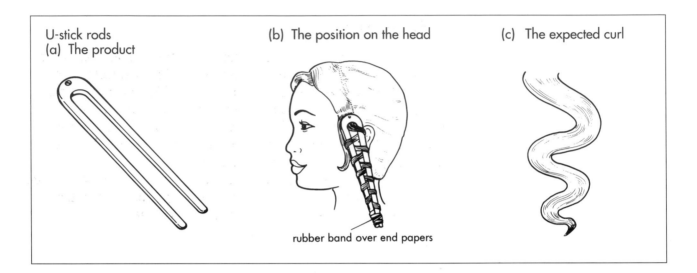

U-stick rods
(a) The product   (b) The position on the head   (c) The expected curl

rubber band over end papers

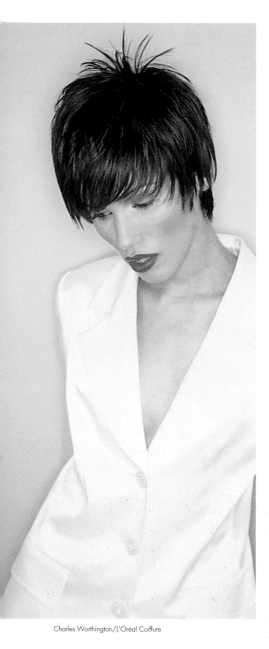

Charles Worthington/L'Oréal Coiffure

CHAPTER 6

Creative colouring

INTRODUCTION

Modifying natural hair colour creates a further dimension to the overall look. It can bring to life many of the internal factors of the hairstyle, as well as the peripheral features. The colours used can either contrast or subtly blend with the natural skin tones and colour of clothes worn. Make-up also contributes to the variety of effects. Lighting, with its reflection and refraction of colours and pigments, further enhances the image.

Within this chapter we provide step-by-step guidance to creative colouring designs, as well as relevant background information. The building blocks you need to consider include:

Shape and form

Lines and angles

Adopted techniques

Apparent texture

Movement and direction

Dimensions, distribution and abundance

Colour depth and tone

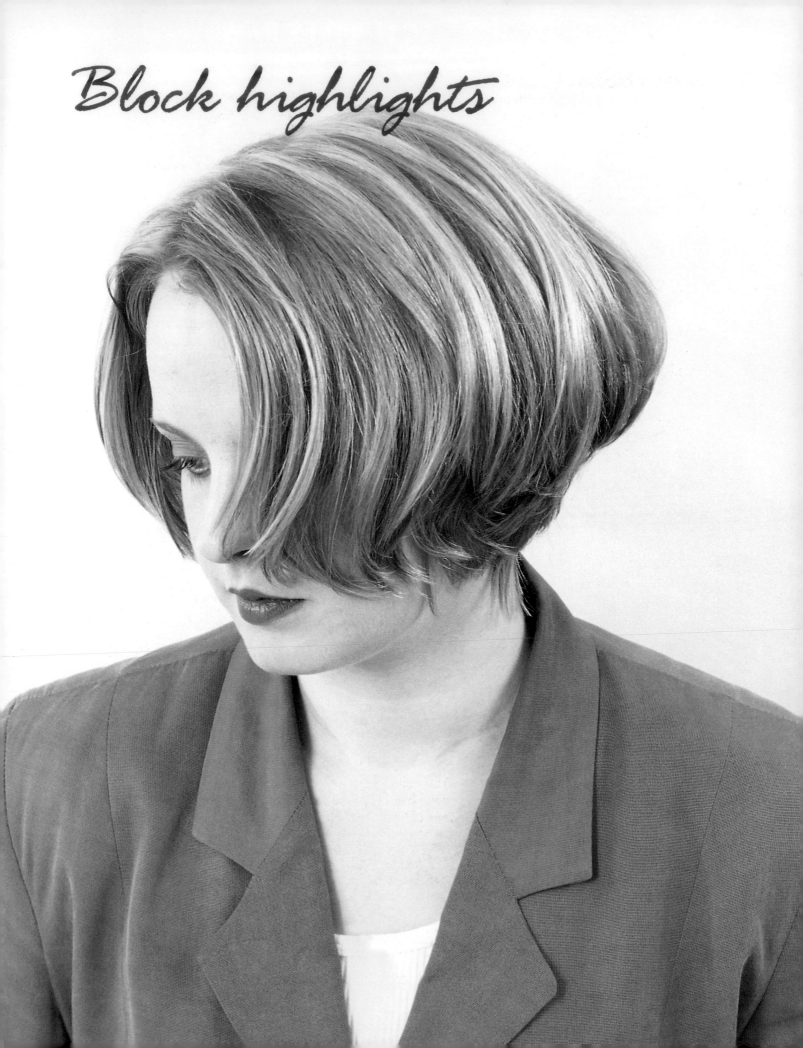

Block highlights

Key building blocks

Shape and form

This simple but attractive hairstyle is achieved using a clever combination of subtle colouring and precision cutting.

Lines and angles

The lines created by colour and movement accentuate the textural effects within the hairstyle as well as the perimeter shape.

Movement and direction

The delicate lines of colour within the shape augment the movement created by the cut.

Colour depth and tone

The soft tones of blonde on blonde enhance the volume and softened edges of the hairstyle.

Step-by-step guidance

The following step-by-step sequence uses Matrix's colour graphics – a lightening product range that allows you to mix lightening powder with a peroxide-based promoter and colour pigment. Six colour pigments are available within the range: three cool (green, blue and violet) and three warm (yellow, orange and red). The pigments are used with the lightener to either neutralise unwanted natural tones within the hair or increase tonal effects.

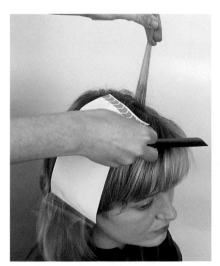

1 Take wide sections of hair (approximately 30 mm by 5 mm) at the parting area.

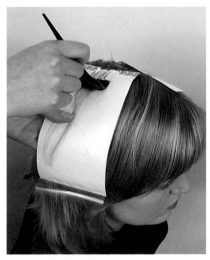

2 Warm yellow colour graphics have been selected for these sections of hair.

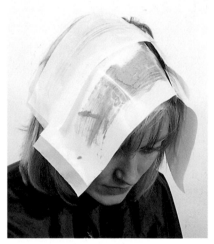

3 Contrasting cool blue colour graphics complete the parting colour.

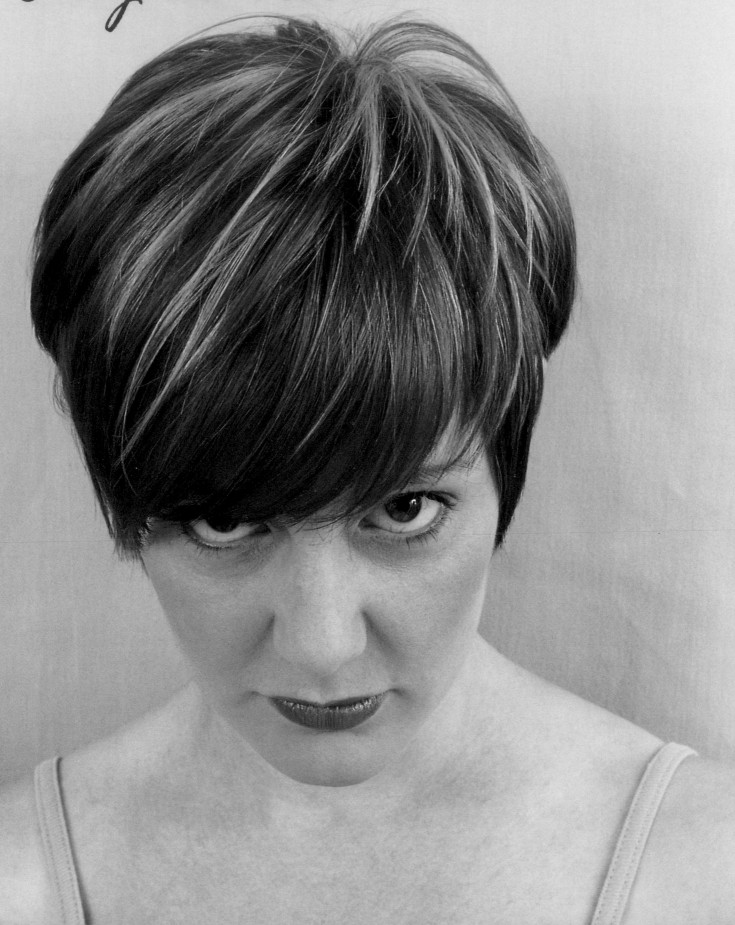

Layered colour

Key building blocks

Shape and form

The positioning of colour within the hair needs to be guided by the natural hair fall.

Lines and angles

The gently curving lines help to achieve balance. The asymmetry created by both the cut lines and the short light hair at the crown contrasts with a low, richly coloured fringe.

Colour depth and tone

Three colours are used to produce a softly contrasting two-tone effect, as opposed to the expected dramatic contrast created between reds and blondes. With this particular look, strong colour with a little light hair around the fringe forms a pleasing focal point.

Step-by-step guidance

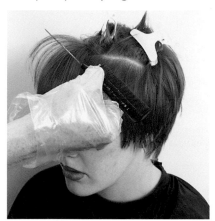

1 First tint the full head of hair. Once this is completed, divide a 30 mm by 2 mm section horizontally at the front.

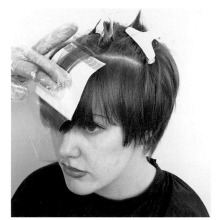

2 Place this section of hair into a colour packet, colour wrap or foil.

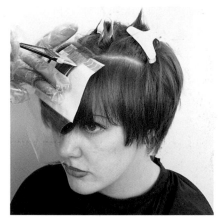

3 Apply a dark brown background tint.

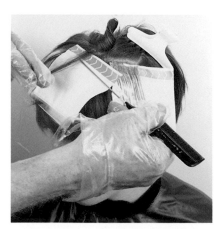

4 Then take narrower sections (5 mm by 5 mm square) to overlie the wider background. Lighten these with a contrasting colour.

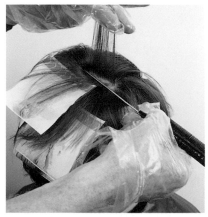

5 Take further sections, working up the head.

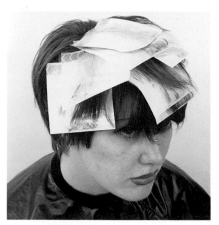

6 Leave the hair until the full colour development takes place.

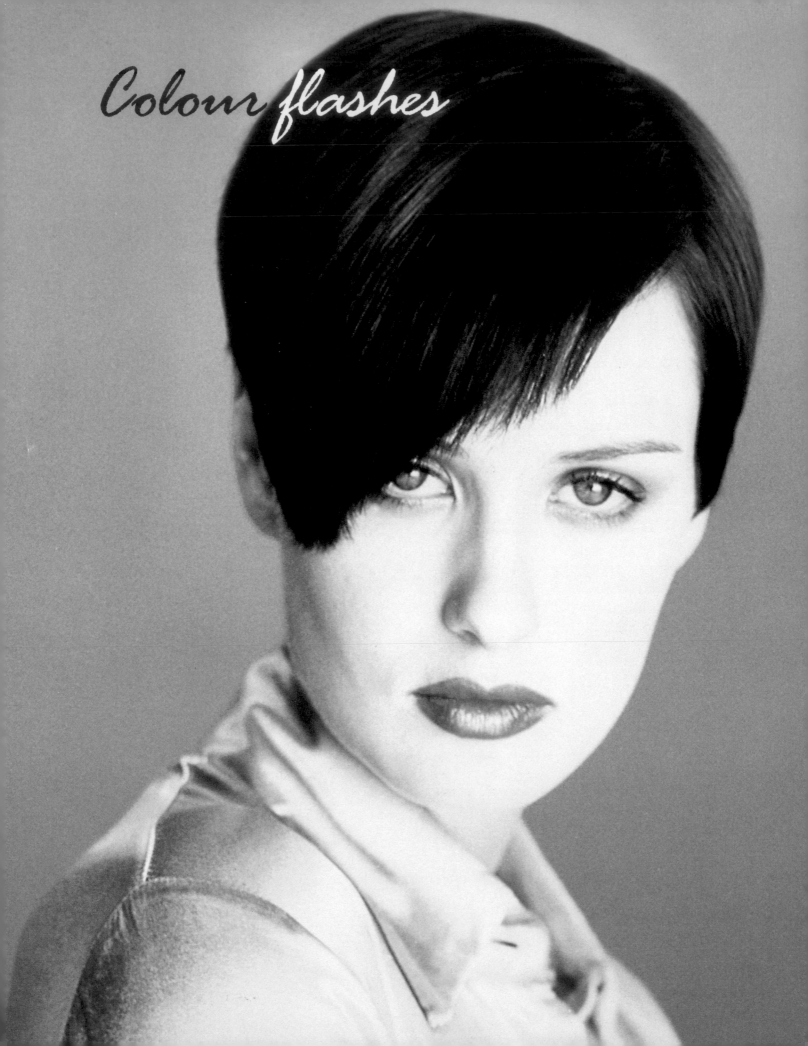

Colour flashes

Key building blocks

Shape and form

This is a chic head-hugging shape, using asymmetry to create a dramatic effect.

Lines and angles

A stark contrast is created between the right and left sides of the face. This asymmetric cut exposes the forehead above one eye, which is balanced by a partial diagonal covering of the other eye.

Colour depth and tone

This is a good example of the use of contrasting effects. The warmth of the colour flash at the side front is countered by the cool eye colour.

Step-by-step guidance

1 After shampooing and conditioning, cut and dry the hair into style. (This is essential for the positioning of the graphic colour effect.)

2 Using the mirror in front of the client, note how the light reflects the curvature of the shape. This helps to locate the exact position of the colour flash.

3 Take sections from either side of the parting from the point at which the light is reflected – approximately 20 mm by 5 mm in width – and place on to colour wraps or something similar.

4 Mix the selected warm shade with the appropriate developer.

5 Apply the colourant to the predetermined point of the hair.

6 Leave the colourant to develop.

7 To complete the overall effect, apply a quasi-tint (e.g. Color Touch) to the remaining hair and leave to develop.

8 After removing the colourant, blow dry the hair into style.

9 Any remaining harsh lines of colour may be removed by personalising the effect with the gentle use of a razor or shaper.

Asymmetric shimmer

Key building blocks

Shape and form

A dramatic effect is produced by the full weight at the hair points; this contemporary style is a reflection of a classic 1960s bob.

Lines and angles

The cut line is stark and blunt. This is due in part to the straightness of the hairstyle. The frontal area is softened by tucking the hair behind the ears and an asymmetrical section is allowed to fall forward.

Colour depth and tone

The lighter, warmer contrasting colour is positioned asymmetrically: the inner-lying hair is partially coloured on one side, and the surface outer hair is coloured on the other.

Step-by-step guidance

1 After shampooing and conditioning, cut and dry the hair into style. (This is essential for the positioning of the graphic colour effect.)

2 Divide a low parting in the hair.

3 Take a section underneath and behind the ear after pinning the hair bulk out of the way. Subdivide this into three or four strands of coloured hair.

4 On the opposite side of the parting, take a wide, thin mesh of hair (80 mm by 3 mm) and lay it on to a colour wrap.

5 Apply the colourant and leave to develop.

6 Remove the colourant and blow dry the hair into style.

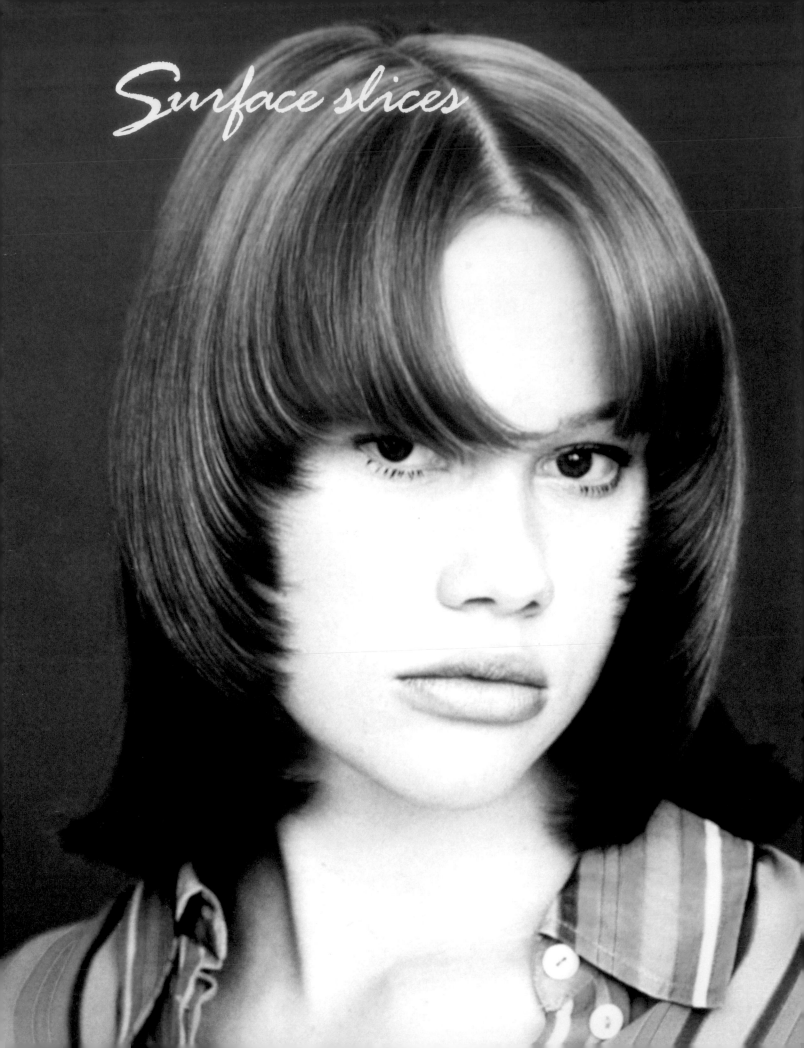

Surface slices

Key building blocks

Shape and form

This symmetrical look is created and emphasised by the dramatic treatment of the hair points when cut. The soft hair touching the cheeks and eyes focuses the evenness of the model's facial features.

Lines and angles

The line of the style curves evenly around the head, falling from a central parting and effectively cloaking the sides.

Colour depth and tone

The style line is augmented by alternating the strands of coloured hair. The warmth of the hair complements the warmth of the eyes.

Step-by-step guidance

1 First tint the whole head of hair to provide the background colour.

2 After shampooing and conditioning, cut and dry the hair into style. (This is essential for the positioning of the graphic colour effect.)

3 Take sections up to 20 mm by 3 mm at the parting area and put them into colour wraps. Apply a suitable lightener. Note the fineness of the sections – only a few millimetres in depth – which ensures that they merge with the background colour.

4 After the lightener has developed, remove it at the basin in the usual way.

5 Then dry the hair into position. Complete the effect by texturising the hair points.

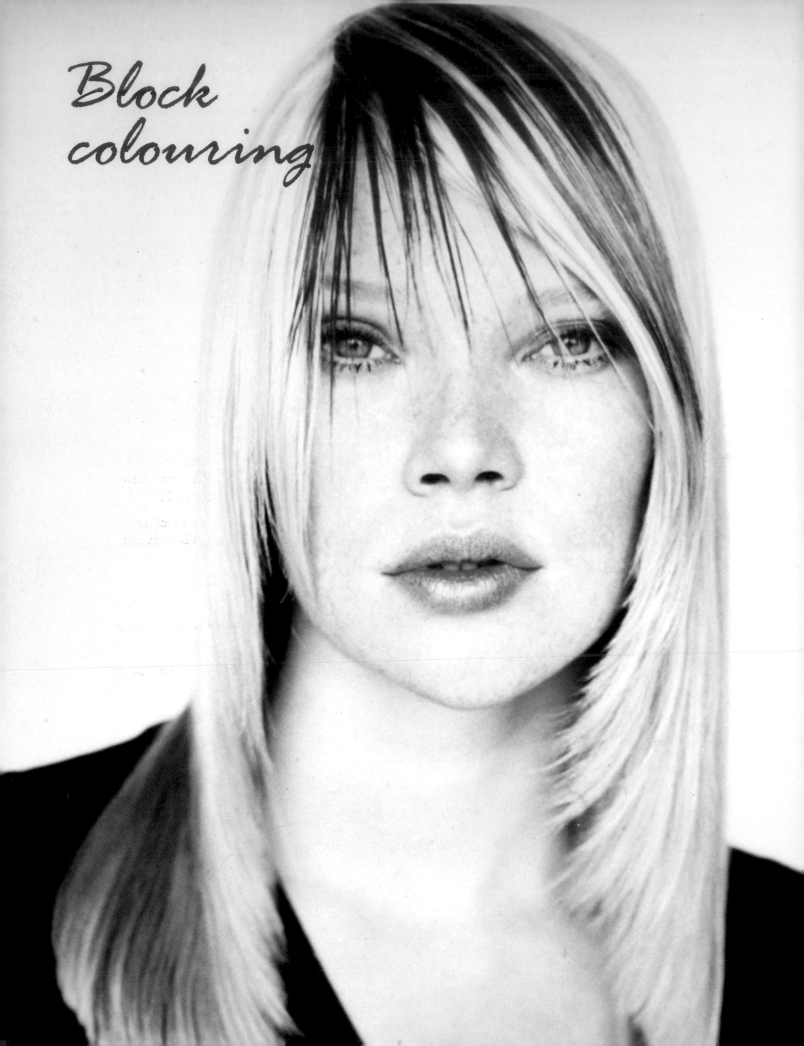

Block
colouring

Key building blocks

Shape and form

The shape of the style is produced by the hair falling from the top section around the face and neck. The hair length is retained and the hair points are dramatically texturised.

Lines and angles

The line of the style is emphasised by the alternating coloured strands with the contrast of coloured frontal hair. This sweeping, curving effect is due to both the cut line and complementing colours.

Colour depth and tone

The darker frontal spikes of hair contrast with the lighter curving hair swirling towards the front. This highlights the delicate balance of the facial features. The eye colour and surrounding colour of the eye make-up produce an effective image.

Step-by-step guidance

1 After shampooing and conditioning, cut and dry the hair into style. (This is essential for the positioning of the graphic colour effect.)

2 Take a triangular section, with one edge following the parting line and the other edge diagonally passing to a position above the eye. This provides the perimeter for the fringe colour.

3 Take a fine mesh along the parting and secure it to the other side of the head. This provides the overfall of some blonde hair in the final effect.

4 Tint the rest of the triangular section.

5 After the colourant has developed, remove it in the usual way at the basin.

6 Add texture to the fringe with the use of a razor and final scissor pointing.

7 Dry the hair into style to achieve the completed effect.

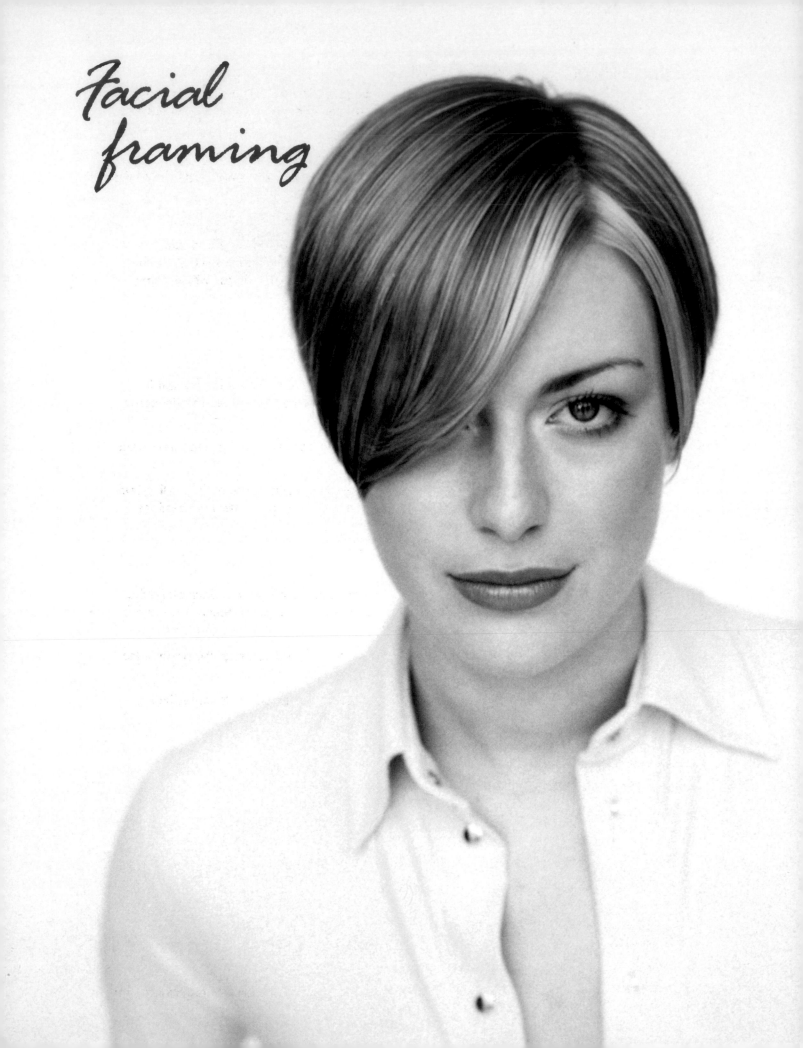

Facial framing

Mahogany

Key building blocks

Shape and form

The clear form of the hair bulk, with its soft fullness, blends into the face and head shape. The asymmetrical effect produced is striking.

Lines and angles

The direction in which the lines of the hair flow is clear and continuous throughout. This emphasises the balance and adds to the shape of the style.

Colour depth and tone

The hair colour throughout matches the natural eye and skin colouring, and the added colour strands bring the style to life. The lightly coloured strands produce a pleasing softness which brings everything into balanced focus.

Step-by-step guidance

1 After shampooing and conditioning, cut and dry the hair into style. (This is essential for the positioning of the graphic colour effect.)

2 The parting provides the focal point for the lightened front area.

3 Place a section (10 mm by 5 mm) either side of the parting into colour wraps, then do the same with a couple more sections further back on the head.

4 Apply high lift colour or bleach.

5 Then take other fine sections or meshes further back along the parting, place them into wraps and lighten them in the same way.

6 After full development, remove the colourant at the basin in the usual way.

7 Blow dry the hair into style and apply serum to make the hair shine.

COLOURING PRINCIPLES

Hair pigmentation

The natural colour of hair is determined by the colour of pigments within the hair's cortex. These are formed when the hair is in its germinating stage of growth.

Hair colour pigments – *melanin* – are deposited into the hair shaft at the region of the papilla and germinal matrix. The pigments responsible for black and brown hair are called *eumelanin*; those responsible for red and yellow hair are called *pheomelanin*. (There are in fact others, but these are the main pigments.) The hair colour you actually see is affected by the amount and proportion of the pigments present, by the light in which the hair is seen, and – to a certain extent – by the colours of the clothes and make-up worn.

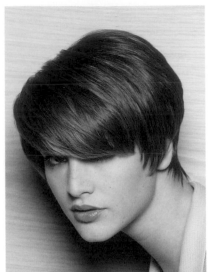

With age, or after periods of stress, the production of natural pigments may be reduced. The hairs already on the head will not be affected, but the new ones will. As hairs fall out and are replaced, the proportion that have the original pigmentation diminishes and the hair's overall colour changes. It may become lighter. If no pigment is produced at all, then the new hairs will be white.

The proportion of white hairs among the naturally coloured ones causes the hair to *appear* grey. Greyness is often referred to as a percentage; for example, '50% grey' means that half of the hairs on the head are white and the rest are pigmented.

It is not uncommon for young people to exhibit some grey hairs – this does not necessarily mean that they will go grey, or completely white, at an early age.

Natural hair colour

The *depth* of colour is a description of how light or dark the colour is. This depends on the intensity of the pigments within the hair.

The *tone* is the colour that you see – the combination of pigments that give the overall colour. 'Warm' shades such as gold or auburn have proportionately more pheomelanin. 'Cool' shades, such as ash, cendre, matt or drab, have less.

The natural hair colour that we see results from the *reflection* of some of the light falling on the hair. White light is actually a combination of many colours. These can be seen separated when the light has passed through a prism or through droplets of rain, giving the familiar colour spectrum of the rainbow: red–orange–yellow–green–blue–indigo–violet. Thus, hair that appears auburn in natural white light is *absorbing* most of the light at the blue–violet end of the spectrum, but *reflecting* much of the light at the red–yellow end.

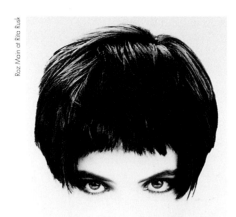

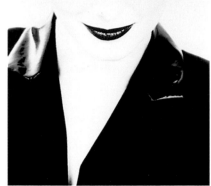

Roz Main at Rita Rusk

Artificial light does not contain the full range of colours that together make up natural white light. This can affect the apparent colour of the hair. If, for example, there is no red in the artificial light, the hair cannot reflect red light and may appear colder in colour. In general:

- the white light of full daylight shows the true hair colour
- the yellowish light given by some bare electric bulbs adds warmth to hair colour, but neutralises blue or ash colour effects
- the bluish light produced by some fluorescent tubes tends to neutralise the warmth of red hair colours.

Artificial or synthetic colour

The colours of tints used on hair are based on the three *primary* pigment colours: red, blue and yellow. When pairs of primary colours are mixed together, the *secondary* colours are produced:

- red + yellow → orange
- yellow + blue → green
- blue + red → purple/violet.

The International Colour Chart defines hair colours systematically. There are some differences between manufacturers in the way that they describe or name colours.

Colour	Depth	Colour	Tone
1/0	blue-black	–/0	natural
2/0	black	–/1	special ash
3/0	dark brown	–/2	cool ash
4/0	medium brown	–/3	honey gold
5/0	light brown	–/4	red/gold
6/0	dark blonde	–/5	purple
7/0	medium blonde	–/6	violet
8/0	light blonde	–/7	brunette
9/0	very light blonde	–/8	pearl ash
10/0	extra light blonde	–/9	soft ash

The International Colour Chart

Shades of colour are numbered, with black (number 1) at one end of the scale and lightest blonde (10) at the other. *Tones* of colour range from 0.1 to 0.9. In combination these yield a large number of colours.

Colour charts usually arrange the colour shades along the side and the tones of colour across the top. To use these charts, first identify the base shade of the client's hair colour, then read along the column to see the different colours that you should be able to produce from that shade. For example, if your client has a base hair shade of light brown hair (shade number 5) and you tint with an orange tone of red/gold (0.4), the result should be a light warm brown (5.4).

There is a large range of colours which you can use to produce a wide variety of effects. Be sure to follow the manufacturer's

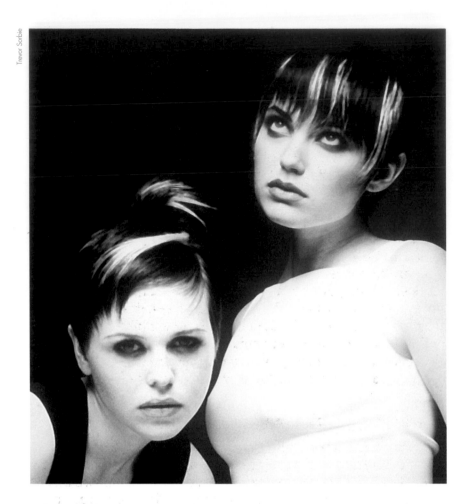

guide for each colour in order to produce their specialist colour ranges.

Note that with natural colour:

- depth depends on the amount of dark/light pigment
- tone depends on the distribution of warm/ash pigment.

With artificial colour, on the other hand:

- all colours are combinations of primary and secondary colours
- opposite colours of the colour circle neutralise each other.

HAIR COLOURANTS

Temporary colourants

Temporary colourants are available in the form of lotions, creams, mousses, gels, lacquers, sprays, crayons, paints and glitterdust. On hair in good condition these do not penetrate the hair cuticle, nor do they directly affect the natural hair colour, they simply remain on the hair until washed off.

Temporary colourants are ideal for a client who has not had colour before, as they are readily removed if not liked. They have subtle colouring effects, particularly on grey or greying hair. Hair condition, shine and control are enhanced.

If used on badly damaged or very porous hair, the temporary colourant may quickly be absorbed into the cortex, producing uneven, patchy results.

Semi-permanent colourants

Semi-permanent colourants are made in a variety of forms – some ready-mixed for immediate use, others needing to be mixed and prepared as necessary before use. Always check the manufacturer's instructions to ensure that you know which type of colourant you are going to use.

Semi-permanent colourants contain pigments which are deposited in the hair cuticle and outer cortex. The colour gradually lifts each time the hair is shampooed. Some colourants will last through six washes, others longer.

These colourants are not intended to cover large percentages of white hair – for instance, black used on white hair would not produce a pleasing result. Choose colours carefully.

Note that some permanent colourants may be diluted for use as semi-permanents. These products may contain skin sensitisers, however, so skin tests must be performed before use in this way.

Longer-lasting colourants

Now that 'frequent use' shampoos have become popular, some semi-permanent colourants are soon removed. A new generation of longer-lasting colourants has been introduced which are more practical and economical. These colourants allow for a greater coverage of white hair, and last for up to 12 washes.

Quasi-permanent colourants

These colourants are nearly permanent – they last for a longer period of time than semi-permanent colourants but not as long as the true permanent colourants. When using them, follow the manufacturer's instructions strictly.

Permanent colourants

Permanent colourants are made in a wide variety of shades and tones. They can cover white and natural-coloured hair to produce a range of natural, fashion and fantasy shades.

Hydrogen peroxide is mixed with permanent colourants. This oxidises the hair's natural pigments and joins the small molecules of synthetic pigment together, a process called *polymerisation*. The hair will then retain the colour permanently in the cortex. Hair in poor condition, however, will not hold the colour and colouring could result in patchy areas and colour fading.

The use of modern permanent colourants can lighten or darken the natural hair colour, or both together in one process. This is achieved by varying the percentage strength of hydrogen peroxide.

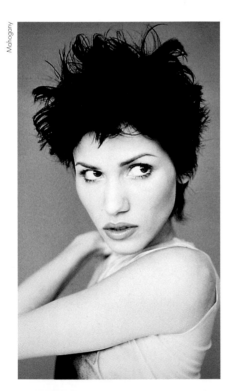

Mahogany

HEALTH AND SAFETY

Before using permanent colourants, you must perform a skin test. If there is a positive reaction, do not carry out the tinting: to do so could result in an allergic reaction.

Colour choice

Your choice of colour is crucial: take time to make it carefully. A hurried choice may give disastrous results!

A number of questions need to be answered before the final choice of colour is made.

What does the client require?

Commonly clients requesting a permanent colour are seeking to disguise their greying hair. A client who wants something to tone a few grey hairs may be successfully assisted with temporary, semi-permanent or longer-lasting colourants. However, if the client is really longing simply to be young again it is difficult to help much with any type of colour, though it may well be possible to help her to look a little more youthful.

If the colouring is intended for a special occasion, the colour of the clothes to be worn, the colour of the make-up to be used, and the colour of the surroundings – lighting, wallcoverings and so on – will all have their effect on the colour reflected on to the client's face and hair, and hence on the *apparent* colour of the hair. These points should be considered before deciding which shade of permanent colourant to apply.

What other factors are relevant?

During your consultation with your client, you will need to consider the following points:

- the client's age and lifestyle
- her job, if she has one
- her fashion and dress sense, and the colours she prefers to wear
- her natural hair colour and her skin colour
- the hair's texture, condition and porosity
- the colourant you could use
- the time and cost involved.

When you have taken these points into consideration, you should be able to determine which hair colour shade, colourant and process to recommend to your client.

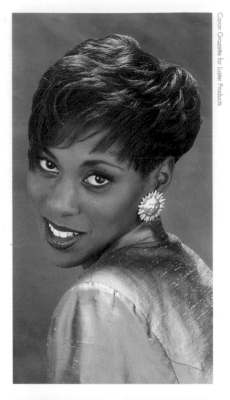

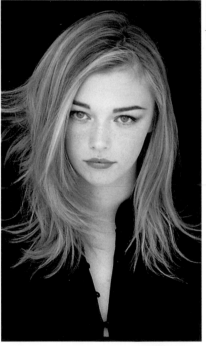

Colouring: problems and solutions

Problem	Possible causes	Solution
Patchy results	Insufficient tint coverage Poor application Colour mix poor Sections too large Overlapped tint Underprocessed tint Spirit-based products used	Spot tint light areas Reduce dark areas Apply toners to neutralise colours Double-check condition of hair
Colour too light	Wrong colour shade chosen Peroxide strength too low Underprocessed Hair too porous Peroxide strength too high	Recondition hair Colour-fill if necessary Use darker shade Test to assess correct peroxide strength
Colour fade after two or three shampoos	Sun-bleached Underprocessed Rough physical treatment Hair too porous	Recondition Apply dilute colour Avoid repeatedly combing undiluted tint through hair
Colour too dark	Wrong colour chosen Overprocessed Hair too porous Incompatible colour present	Apply colour reducer Follow manufacturer's instructions
Hair too red	Peroxide strength too high Wrong neutralising colour used Incomplete development Hair underbleached	Apply matt/green to neutralise
Hair discoloured	Hair too porous Hair not holding colour Possibly coated with incompatibles If green, blue may have been used on yellow base, or there may be a metallic salt reaction If mauve, possible chemical reaction with an incompatible substance	Correct green with red, but beware of producing dark brown Correct mauve with yellow, If necessary, apply colour reducers
Good general coverage except for white hair	Hair was too resistant Not enough base shade used	Pre-soften white hair Apply base shade direct to white hair
Hair generally too resistant to tint	Tight cuticle Underprocessed Incorrect colour choice Poor mixing or application	Pre-soften hair Time reapplication accurately Select colour carefully Mix tint thoroughly Apply as recommended
Scalp reaction	Hair not washed thoroughly Peroxide strength too high Rough combing and application Allergic reaction has occurred	If minor irritation, ensure cleanliness of scalp If scalp is broken, swelling or painful, give no further salon treatment and send client to the doctor; notify salon's insurance company

Tests

Don't forget that the following tests are designed to help you and to protect your client:

- *skin test* – to assess the client's sensitivity to the tint
- *colour test* – to assess the suitability of the chosen colour
- *porosity test* – to assess the smoothness or roughness of the cuticle
- *elasticity test* – to determine the hair's state or condition
- *incompatibility test* – if metallic chemicals are present
- *strand test* – to check the process of colouring.

Make sure that you refer to the client's record card if she has been to the salon before, or make out a new card to note down what you decide and the results of any tests.

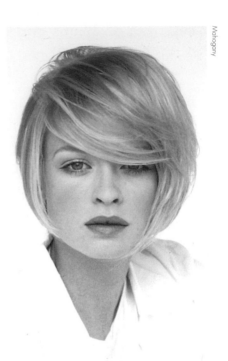

> **HEALTH AND SAFETY**
> Manufacturers' instructions for the use of their products must always be followed to reduce the possibility of damaging or unsatisfactory results.

BLEACHING AND LIGHTENING

Bleaching is a process of making the hair colour lighter. The colour pigment eumelanin is the first to be acted upon; this affects the black and brown colouring. More difficult to alter is pheomelanin, which gives red and yellow colouring. Just how light you can bleach hair is determined by the proportions of the colour pigments present in the hair.

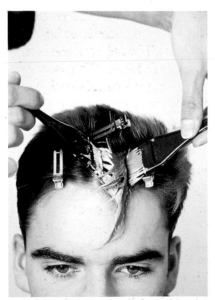

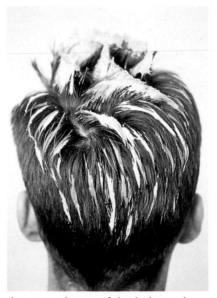

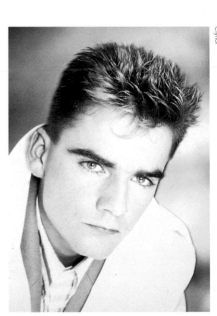

Slices of colour
(a) Applying colour to a sliced section

(b) Completion of the lightened slices

(c) The finished effect

As bleaching proceeds, the hair becomes lighter and lighter. The hair changes colour:

black→brown→red brown→orange→yellow→
light yellow→very light yellow

To check how light you can bleach the hair, take a cutting of the client's hair and apply bleach to it. By careful timing and processing, you should be able to find out exactly how much the hair can take and what colour you can bleach it to. Remember that if the hair contains a lot of red/yellow pigment, it must not be lightened too much – the hair's breaking point will quickly be reached.

The chemistry of bleaching

The chemical process of bleaching is one of *oxidation*: oxygen is added to the chemical pigments. Various types of bleach will do this; *hydrogen peroxide* (H_2O_2) is one of the most common.

Hydrogen peroxide is available in cream, foam and liquid forms. It acts in stages. First the bleaching agent causes the hair to swell: the cuticle begins to lift. The bleach can then penetrate to the hair cortex, where the liberated oxygen acts on the pigment, lightening the hair.

Longer times or stronger bleaches may be required for hair of different colours. Just how long is required, and what strength of bleach must be used, can be determined using a test cutting.

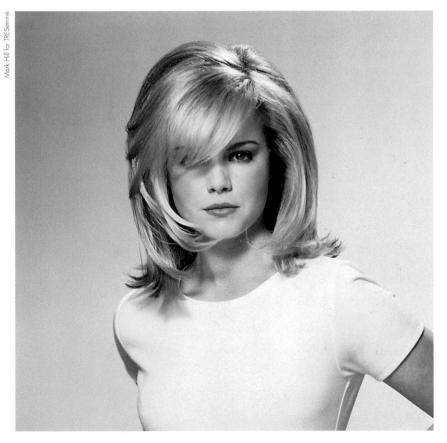

Mark Hill for TRESemmé

Activating the bleach

Hydrogen peroxide is very reactive – it readily produces oxygen – so it needs to be *stabilised* if its effectiveness is to be maintained. This is done by adding chemicals such as sulphuric or phosphoric acids when the bleach is manufactured.

To activate the stabilised hydrogen peroxide, you first need to neutralise the stabilisers. This is done by adding ammonium hydroxide, sodium acetate or ammonium carbonate: you mix these bleach products together. Remember to read and follow the manufacturer's instructions carefully when using bleach products.

Calculating hydrogen peroxide strengths

1 Suppose you start with 30% hydrogen peroxide but want 6%:

$\frac{6}{30} = \frac{1}{5}$ which means that in 5 parts, 1 part should be hydrogen peroxide and therefore 4 parts should be water.

2 To dilute 30% hydrogen peroxide to 18%:

$\frac{18}{30} = \frac{3}{5}$ which means 3 parts hydrogen peroxide to 2 parts water.

3 To dilute 30% hydrogen peroxide to 12%:

$\frac{12}{30} = \frac{2}{5}$ which means 2 parts hydrogen peroxide to 3 parts water.

4 To dilute 30% hydrogen peroxide to 9%:

$\frac{9}{30} = \frac{3}{10}$ which means 3 parts hydrogen peroxide to 7 parts water.

5 To dilute 30% hydrogen peroxide to 3%:

$\frac{3}{30} = \frac{1}{10}$ which means 1 part hydrogen peroxide to 9 parts water.

A *peroxometer* can be used to check hydrogen peroxide strengths.

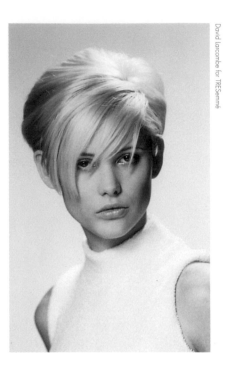

David Larcombe for TRESemmé

Overbleaching

Too much bleaching will destroy the hair's structure. Even if the hair doesn't actually break, it can become spongy, porous or patchy in colour. Further chemical processing – colouring, toning, perming or general hair management – is then very difficult. When wet, overbleached hair stretches like chewing gum and the effects of blow styling or setting cannot last. If hair ever reaches this state, it needs to be treated very gently and conditioned; all harsh processes must be avoided.

Some causes of overbleaching

- The hydrogen peroxide solution was too strong.
- Processing was too long.
- Hair sections overlapped.
- Bleach was repeatedly combed through previously bleached hair.
- The hair was in too poor a condition at the outset, and was very porous.
- The hair had been overexposed to sun, wind, sea or chlorinated water.

The choice of bleach

Explore fully the range of bleach products that are available: make sure that you are confident about their use and effects.

For each client, carefully consider the bleaching process and determine which techniques will be helpful. Here are some guidelines:

- Consult the client and ascertain her wishes.
- Discuss the various possibilities.
- Examine the client's hair and scalp; determine what is possible.
- Consider the client's natural base colour.
- Determine what colouring, if any, has already been used on the hair.
- Consider the client's eyes and facial colour, and find out what colours she likes to wear.
- Is the colouring appropriate to the client's lifestyle?
- Make a skin test, if necessary.
- Test a sample cutting of the hair.
- Agree with your client exactly what is to be done.

COLOUR VARIATIONS

There are many ways of bleaching and toning your client's hair apart from a whole-head bleach process or the usual regrowth application. The hair can be:

- *highlighted* – colour can be applied or lightened in contrasting streaks or areas
- *lowlighted* – colour can be applied or lightened in streaks or areas, matched more closely to the general colour
- *tipped, frosted, striped or vari-coloured* – names given to various degrees and techniques of lightening or toning parts of the hair
- *shaded* without lightening – for instance, adding darker or warmer shades to naturally fair hair, or burgundy/plum shades to brown hair.

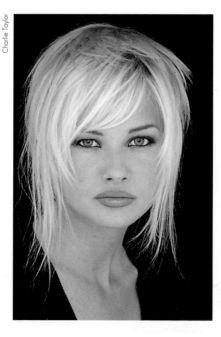
Charlie Taylor

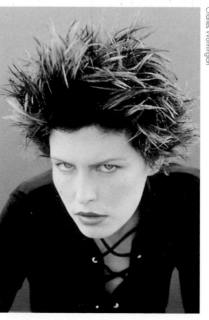
Charles Worthington

There are endless variations – small blocks of lightened or toned hair, a few streaks or stripes, lightly tipped parts to highlight a style line, and so on. Often the more natural, softer, blending tones are the most pleasing, but contrasting tones can be very effective. Check the instructions from your colour manufacturer and take account of their specialist recommendations.

You need to be clear exactly how much and which parts of the hair you are going to lighten. The style worn should help to determine the parts to be bleached. Your proposals should, of course, be fully discussed and agreed with your client.

Methods of bleaching and colouring

To achieve the variety of effects possible, there are several ways in which you can make the bleach or colour application. Always follow manufacturers' instructions on how to use their products. Examples are:

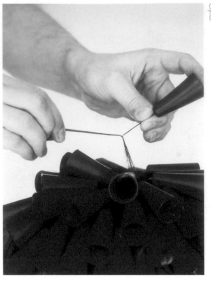
Colouring cups

- *Colouring cups* Small plastic containers in which the bleach or colour can be safely contained.
- *Dappling* A popular means of using bleach or colour to produce varied effects.
- *Aluminium foil* This can be ideal for firmly wrapping bleached or coloured parcels of hair. Different coloured foils can be used to identify different areas and colours used.
- *Highlight caps* Basic 'lighting' resources, which can be used to achieve advanced effects such as multi-lighting, spot lighting or varitoning.
- *Colour wraps* These make it easier to process slices, sections or parcels of bleached or coloured hair safely.
- *Section and pin* A method of selecting areas of the hair to be coloured by shaping them into curl formations and pinning them into position.

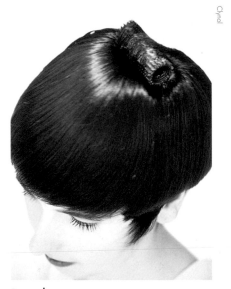
Dappling

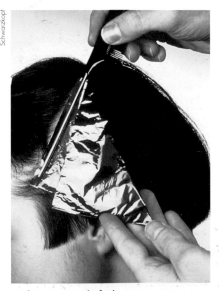

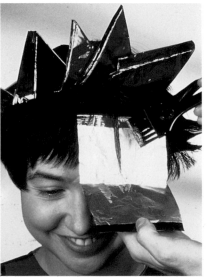
Colouring with foil

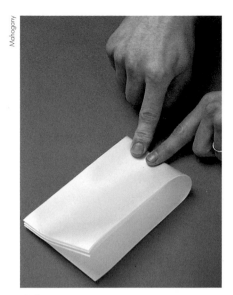

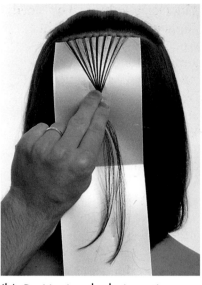

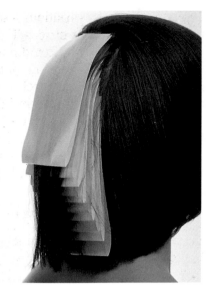

Colour wraps
(a) The product

(b) Positioning the hair section

(c) A completed back panel

In choosing a process, bear in mind that bleach must remain firmly in contact with the hair, but it must not be allowed to run out on to the scalp. Sectioning and sub-sectioning of the parcels of hair must be reasonably convenient for you to carry out.

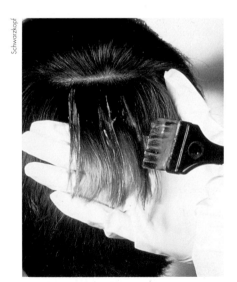

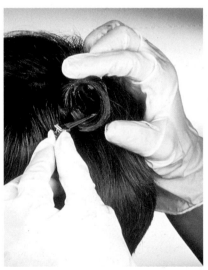

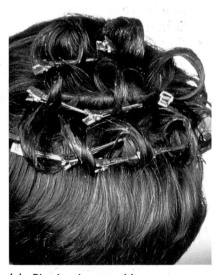

Section and pin
(a) Sectioning and applying colour

(b) Forming the curl

(c) Pinning into position

RECOLOURING

When recolouring bleached hair back to its original or a darker colour, you need to consider the condition of the hair – how porous it might be, and whether there is sufficient colour pigment left in the hair for the hair to retain new pigment.

To ensure that recolouring is successful, it is usual to *pre-pigment* (colour-fill) the hair, applying red or warm shades before the final shade is applied. If this is not done the hair may fade, become patchy or appear greenish. Pre-pigmenting may use temporary, semi-permanent, longer-lasting or permanent colourants.

TONING

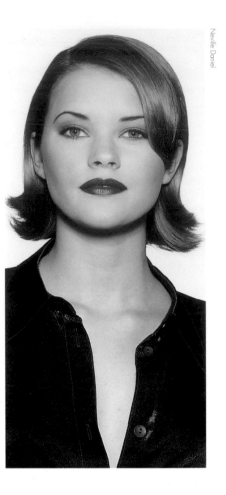

Toning is the process of adding colour to previously bleached or lightened hair. A variety of pastel shades, such as beige, silver and rose are used to produce subtle effects. Different types of toners are available; read the instructions provided by their manufacturers to find out what is possible.

The lightest toners can be used only on the lightest bleached hair: if the hair is too dark, it will absorb the toner colour. Adding colour to colour produces a slightly darker shade of the previous colour.

Mixing colours together produces a wide range of new colours. The following are a few examples:

- red + green → brown
- red + yellow → orange
- blue + yellow → green
- blue + red → violet.

Also:

- red neutralises green
- blue neutralises orange
- violet neutralises yellow.

The *final* colour depends on both the base shade and the toners used.

Toning: problems and solutions

As with any other chemical process, toning problems can be corrected only if the hair and scalp condition permit.

Problem	Possible causes	Action
Uneven colour	Poor application	Spot-bleach
	Section too large	Recolour
	Incorrect mixing	Strip colour and recolour if necessary
Dark ends	Ends underbleached	Rebleach
	Toners too dark	Remove using lighteners
	Toner overprocessed	After removal, time accurately
	Dark tint remains	Remove and tone
Too yellow	Underbleached	Rebleach
	Base too dark	Try stronger bleach
	Wrong toner used	Use violet toner
	Wrong bleach	Use other than oil bleach
Too red	Underbleached	Rebleach
	Too much alkali	Use different bleach
	Wrong toner used	Use green matt or olive

Problem	Possible causes	Action
Dark roots or patches	Poor application Toner too dark	Rebleach evenly Remove using lightener
Roots not coloured	Underbleached Undertimed Toner too dilute Unclean or coated	Rebleach Rebleach Reapply Clean and reapply
Colour fade	Overporous Harsh treatment Overexposure Overprocessed	Condition Advise on hair care Keep hair covered Comb through with diluted colour only
Hair breakage	Overprocessed Incompatibles present Harsh treatment Sleeping in rollers	Recondition remaining hair Test to make sure Give hair-care advice Show effects and avoid
Discolouration	Underprocessed Excessive exposure Home treatments	Colour match or develop further after testing for incompatibles Recondition hair and keep covered Check and advise
Green tones	Incompatibles Blue used on yellow Too-blue ash used	Test hair Use warm or red shades Use violet
Too orange	Underprocessed Pigment lacking	Apply blue or ash Add blue
Too yellow	Underprocessed	Add violet and/or bleach further
Hair tangled	Overbleached Poor shampooing Backcombing remains	Use anti-oxidents; condition Use correct movements Remove and demonstrate
Inflammation	Skin reaction Torn scalp Disease	Do not treat further: seek doctor's advice Seek medical treatment Seek doctor's advice
Irritation	Skin reaction Harsh treatment Disease	Seek doctor's advice Seek doctor's advice Seek doctor's advice
Colour not taking	Overporous Condition poor Pigment lacking Chemicals coating hair	Recondition or colour-fill Recondition Pre-pigment and recolour Remove and recolour
Colour build-up	Overporous Condition poor	Recondition and pre-pigment Recondition
Hair 'stretchy'	Overprocessed* Overporous* Condition very poor*	Condition and treat carefully Recondition Recondition
Hair breaking	Overprocessed† Overlapping† Combing through too much† Incompatibles present†	Recondition remaining hair Recondition Use diluted tint only Test

*Do not attempt to process any further or the hair is likely to break.
†Little can be done when hair has reached this stage other than gentle treatment and conditioning.

DECOLOURING

Decolouring is the process of removing synthetic colourants from the hair. It is also called *colour stripping* or *colour reducing*. Some manufacturers make specific decolouring products – colour strippers or colour reducers – for the removal of their own brands of oxidation tints.

Compound henna and vegetable and mineral dyes can be removed only with special colour reducers. Do not use hydrogen peroxide on these: it is incompatible.

HEALTH AND SAFETY

Recolouring after decolouring should take account of the products used. In general, it is wise not to chemically process the hair again after decolouring; but with some products immediate recolouring *is* recommended. Do not attempt to perm decoloured hair for at least a week.

The manufacturers of colouring, bleaching, toning and decolouring products have excellent advisory services: you should acquaint yourself with these. It is vital that you read and keep the instructions for use of their products, and follow their specific recommendations.

ASSIGNMENT

With the permission of your manager, carry out a work-based assignment in which you produce materials for use in your portfolio.

For this assignment you will need to provide sketches and/or photographs with explanatory notes for the following colouring processes:

- lightening hair (both by bleaching and by colour reduction)
- darkening previously lightened hair
- combination colour effects.

After carrying out each of the practical tasks listed above, write explanatory illustrated notes to show:

1 how the final effects were achieved
2 the variety of tools, equipment and products used
3 the effects and potential effects of porosity on the finished results
4 the problems that occurred, and the potential problems that *might* have occurred, and what remedial action is appropriate in each case
5 the relevant health, safety and hygiene requirements.

You may prefer not to compile sketches, photographs and accompanying notes, but instead to video the entire practical tasks and then to give a personal account of what has taken place. Make sure that you address points 1–5 within your account.

QUESTIONS

After completing the assignment, answer these questions in your portfolio.

1 Describe the chemical process of applying permanent synthetic colourants. What precautions should be taken?
2 Describe the chemical process of lightening or bleaching. What precautions should be taken?
3 List the different ways of using combination colouring techniques. What precautions should be taken?
4 How would you choose a suitable colouring, lightening or darkening process for your client?
5 What are the different tests that can or should be used in colouring, lightening and toning?

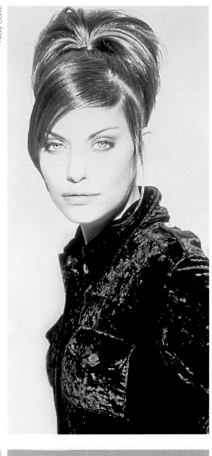

Nicky Clarke

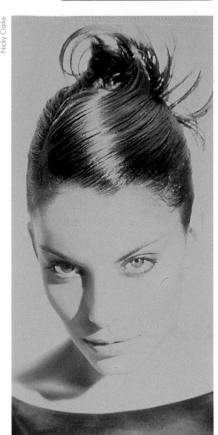

Nicky Clarke

CHAPTER 7

Creative styling and dressing

INTRODUCTION

Clients with long hair may have it dressed into a wide variety of attractive special effects. Some people with shorter hair will want to have hair added to make such styles possible.

A salon specialist will be able to produce a variety of dressed results, starting from a range of different hair lengths. You will already be familiar with the principles of consultation, setting and basic dressing techniques: this chapter looks at methods and applications beyond clients' everyday requirements.

Dressing involves creating special effects and special styles, some of which may be required for particular occasions only. It may entail adding hair, such as hairpieces, wigs or hair extensions. Dressing may also require the imaginative use of ornaments such as combs, slides or headdresses.

Within this chapter we provide step-by-step guidance to a variety of special dressing effects, as well as relevant background information. The building blocks you need to consider include:

Shape and form

Lines and angles

Adopted techniques

Apparent texture

Movement and direction

Dimensions, distribution and abundance

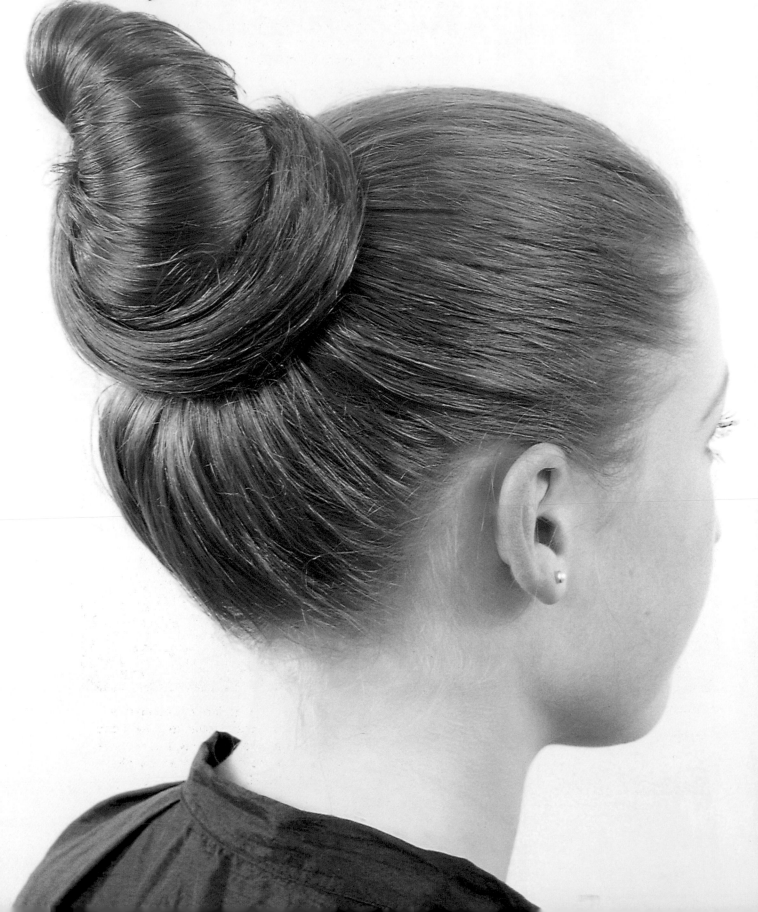

High knot

Key building blocks

Shape and form

The position of the high knot centralises the hair weight at the crown, adding height to the overall image.

Lines and angles

The lines of the hair move directly up from the nape and sides and contrast with the lateral movements of the knot. The position of the knot is determined by the cranial structure and facial features.

Movement and direction

The clean line that the hair takes, with its simple movement, emphasises the structure and proportions of the head and neck.

Step-by-step guidance

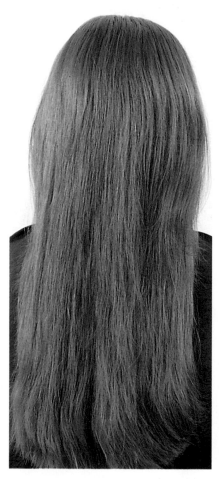

1 Brush and smooth the hair.

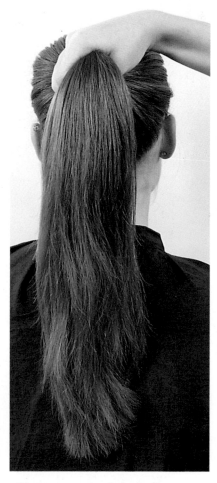

2 Position the hair bulk centrally at the crown and secure.

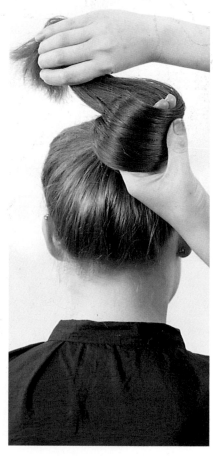

3 Twist the hair at the root end. Continue to twist and turn to the points, first with one hand and then with the other hand. Pin invisibly.

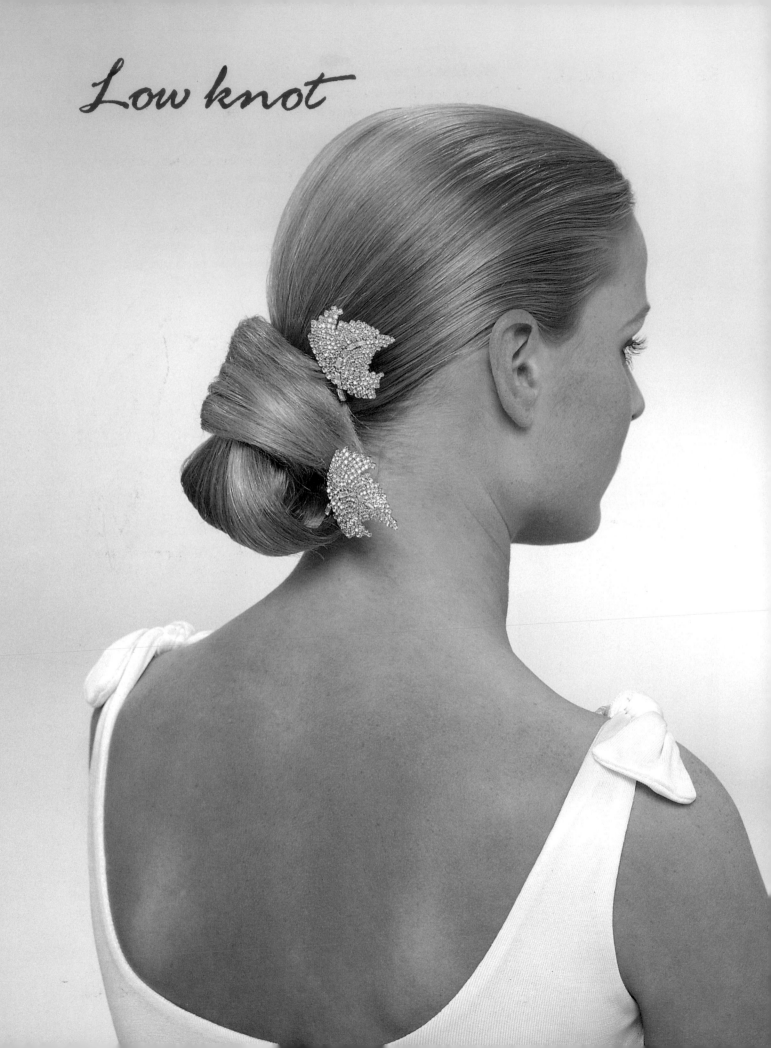

Low knot

Patrick Cameron

Key building blocks

Shape and form

The position of the low knot counterbalances the sleek hair covering the head shape and centralises the hair weight within the nape.

Lines and angles

A dramatic effect is created by the contrast between the vertical line and the crossing of the horizontal fold.

Movement and direction

The clean line that the hair takes, with its simple movement, emphasises the structure of the head and neck.

Step-by-step guidance

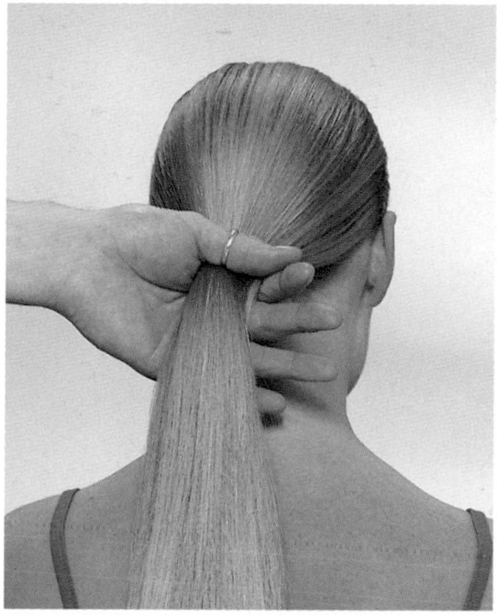

1 Brush the hair and hold it at the nape in a low ponytail. Secure it with a band.

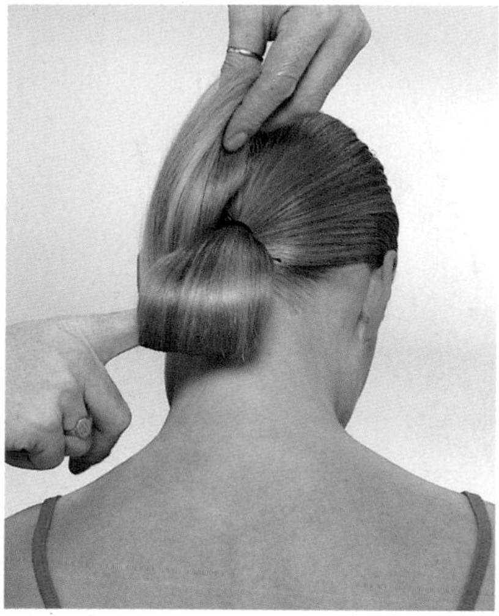

2 Use your finger as a former for the bottom of the knot.

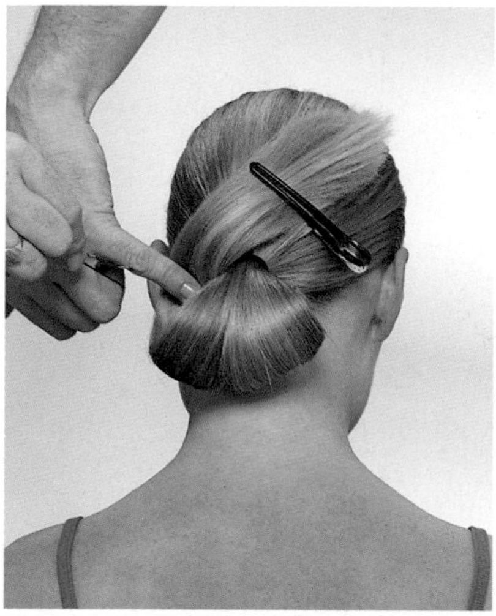

3 Secure the ponytail at one side with grips, while holding the tail hair above.

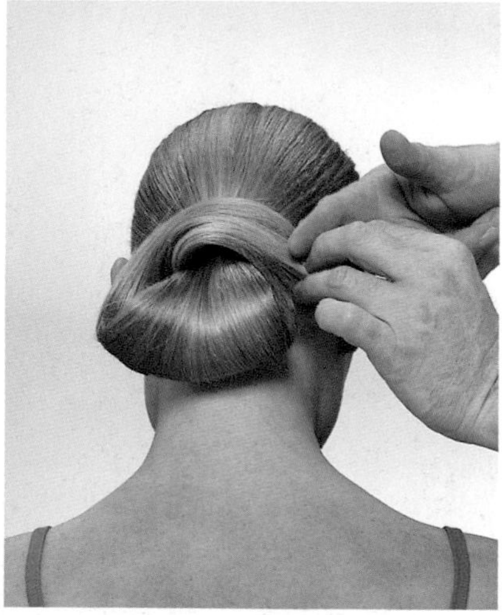

4 Wrap the remaining tail directly across and secure on the other side.

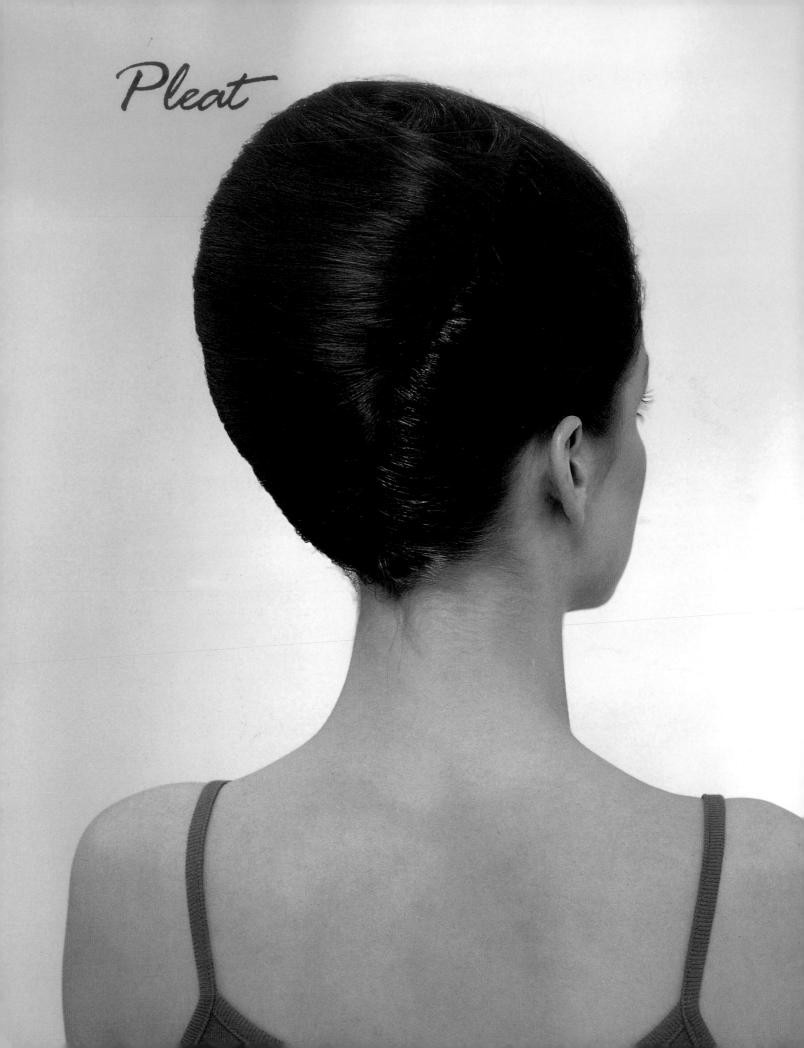

Pleat

Key building blocks

Shape and form

The position of the pleated hair at the back creates interest and emphasises the facial features.

Lines and angles

The line of the hair is smooth or positioned so that it moves from right to left at the back of the head. It is secured firmly into position. The hairline is made to move back from left to right, overriding the base hair which is firmly anchored by grips and pins.

Movement and direction

The curves of the pleat soften the harshness of the contrasting directions within the hair.

Step-by-step guidance

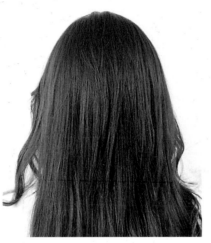

1 Brush the hair to remove any tangles.

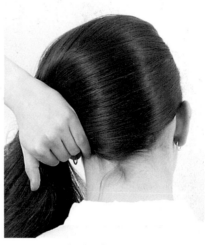

2 Smooth the hair into position, moving the hair back from the face.

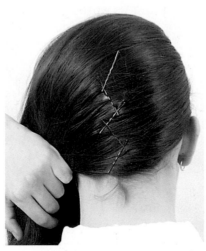

3 Place a row of grips or pins centrally from the nape to the crown.

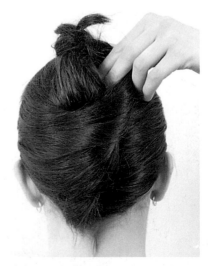

4 Pass the hair over your hand, then grip the hair, turn it and place it in position on the head. Pin the edge of the folded hair invisibly.

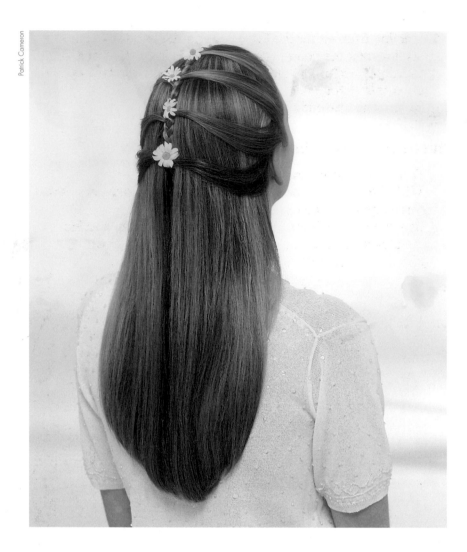

PLAITING

Plaiting is a method of intertwining three or more strands of hair to create a variety of woven hairstyles. When this work is undertaken by the professional stylist for specific occasions, it is often accompanied by ornamentation: fresh flowers and coloured ribbons are popular.

The numerous options for plaited effects are determined by the following factors:

- the number of stems (or plaits) used
- the positioning of the plait or plaits across or around the head
- the way in which the plaits are made (under or over).

Three-stem plait

The three-stem plait is easily achieved and demonstrates the basic principle of plaiting hair.

1 Divide the hair to be plaited into three equal sections.
2 Hold the hair with both hands, using your fingers to separate the sections.

3 Starting from either the left or the right, place the outside section over the centre one. Repeat this from the other side.

4 Continue placing the outside sections of hair over the centre ones until you reach the ends of the stems.

5 Secure the free ends with ribbon or thread.

Three-stem plait – head-hugging style

1 Brush the hair to remove all tangles.

2 With the hair tilted backwards, divide the foremost hair into three equal sections.

3 Starting from either the left or the right, cross an outside stem over the centre stem. Repeat this action with the opposite outer stem.

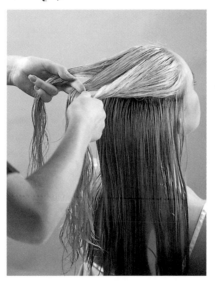

Head-hugging plait
(a) Sectioning the hair

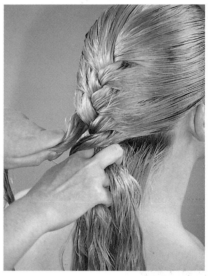

(b) Plaiting the sections in with the main stem

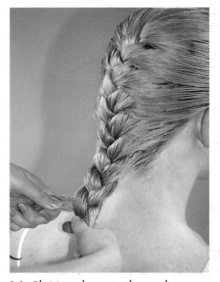

(c) Plaiting down to the ends

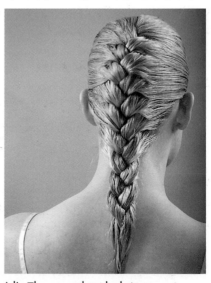

(d) The completed plait

4 Section a fourth stem (less in thickness than the initial three stems) and incorporate this with an outside stem.

5 Cross this thickened stem over the centre, and repeat this step with the opposite outer stem.

6 Continue this sequence of adding hair to the outer stem, before crossing it over the centre.

7 When there is no more hair to be added, continue plaiting down to the ends and secure them.

Four-stem plaits

1 Brush the hair to remove any tangles.

2 Divide the hair to be plaited into four equal stems.

3 Begin to plait by crossing the left-hand centre stem over the right-hand centre stem.

4 Now cross the outside right stem over the stem next to it.

5 Then cross the outside left stem *under* the next one.

6 Repeat steps 3–5 until you reach the hair ends.

Six-stem plaits

1 Brush the hair to remove the tangles.

2 Divide the hair into six equal stems.

3 Pass the outside right stem over the next two stems.

4 From the left, pass the outside stem *under* two stems and *over* one.

5 Repeat this until you reach the hair ends.

Other plaits

- *Using different starting positions* Start plaiting at the side of the head and take the hair around the hairline to produce a halo effect. Or start the plait at the nape, working up the centre of the back and towards the front of the head. Secure the tucked ends with grips to shorten long hair.

- *Under-plaiting* Instead of crossing strands *over* the centre, cross them *under* the centre. This will produce a plait that sits along the head contour.

- *Cornrowing* Divide the hair into small parallel sections and plait it to the scalp. Secure the end of each individual plait with cotton thread. To enhance the effect, decorate the hair with small beads.

WEAVING

Hair weaving is a process of interlacing strands of hair to produce a wide variety of effects. A small area of woven hair can be very effective by itself, or used to highlight a particular part of a style. Hair weaving is also used to place and hold lengths of hair.

At its simplest, hair weaving may be used to hold long hair back from the face. This may be done by taking strands of hair from

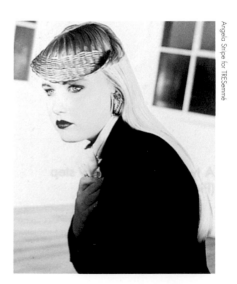

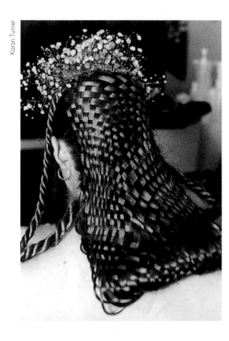

each side, sweeping them over the hair lengths, and intertwining them at the back.

More intricate is the *basket weave* which uses a combination of plaiting, twisting and placing to form many shapes and patterns.

It is important to wet or gel the hair before starting to weave. Weave tightly or loosely according to the effect you are aiming for.

The hair may be woven as follows:

1 Use six meshes of hair, three in the left hand and three in the right.
2 Start with the furthest right-hand mesh. Pass this *over* the inner two meshes.
3 From the left, pass the outside mesh *under* the next two and *over* one.
4 Continue to the ends of the hair.
5 Tuck in the hair ends and secure them in position.

Practise on colleagues or models and experiment with different woven shapes before you attempt to weave hair for clients.

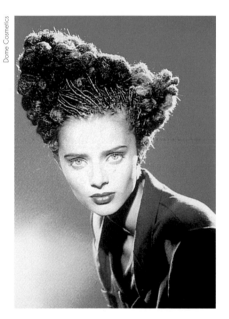

ADDED HAIR – POSTICHE

The addition of hair in the form of postiche – natural or synthetic false hair – has been a feature in many dressings throughout the ages. Postiche has been used to disguise physical injuries and scars, thinning hair and baldness. In dressings it is intended to enhance the overall style, and may take various forms. Here are some examples:

- *Pincurls* are small pieces which you can add to different parts of the dressing. *Ringlets* are larger than pincurls but made and used similarly.
- *Marteaux* are flat, folded pieces of weft attached to the hair by sewn loops or combs. These pieces are useful in adding a wave or waves.
- *Switches* are lengths of weft, spiral-wound or twisted, coiled or plaited in a variety of ways.
- *Torsades* are ornamental twists made from marteaux and switches to form pieces of coiled hair.
- *Swathes*, which may also be made from marteaux and switches, are worn encircling the head. They are useful in securing long hair.
- *Chignons* are rolls or knots worn between the crown and the nape. They are useful in producing additional height, fullness and shape.
- The *cape wiglet* consists of a long length of hair which fits the top of the head and drapes down to the neck. It is used to convert a short head of hair into a longer-looking style. A simple decorative band holds the piece in position.

There are other varieties of postiche, including diamond-mesh foundations, frontal pieces, transformations, scalpettes and full wigs. Each of these has specific uses and may be used as decorative added hair.

Attaching a hairpiece

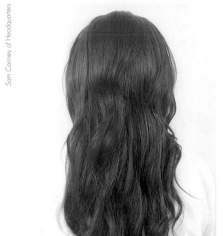

1 Brush the hair to remove any tangles.

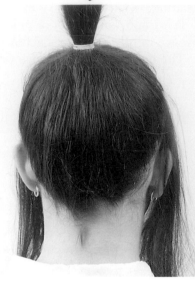

2 Position the hair centrally at the crown and secure.

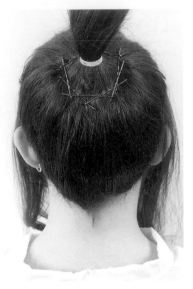

3 An inter-locked base of grips encircles the band on the hair.

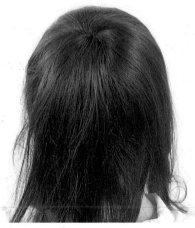

4 Remove the band and spread the hair evenly to provide a secure base.

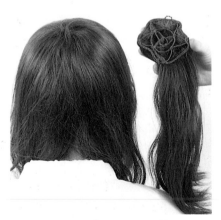

5 The hairpiece ready to be attached.

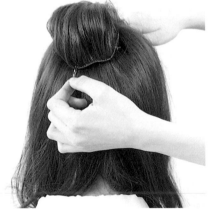

6 The base of the hairpiece is positioned centrally over the crown and gripped into position.

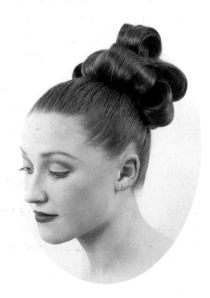

7 Dress the hair as necessary.

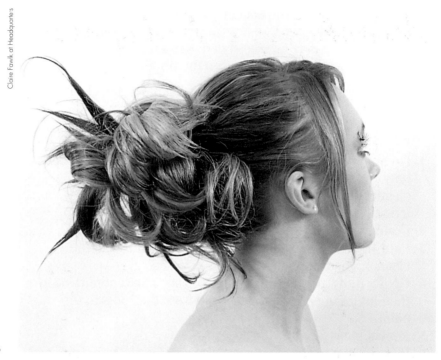

Multiple hairpieces

Care and cleaning

Hairpieces, whether made from real or synthetic hair, must be carefully treated if they are to give good service. To remain hygienic, regular cleaning must be carried out. The more often a hairpiece is worn, the more often it will require cleaning. A wig that is constantly worn should be cleaned at least fortnightly, if not weekly. Care must be taken to avoid damaging the foundation of the hairpiece.

Here are some general points about handling postiche:

- Avoid using sharp combs and brushes which can damage the foundation. Use only the correct dressing techniques.
- Many different synthetic fibres are used in postiche. Follow the manufacturer's instructions for each piece. Synthetic hair may be washed with shampoos.
- Modern synthetic fibres may be set and blow dried; some may even take heated rollers and tonging. If the temperature is too great, however, the curl or wave may be lost.
- Use only those cleaners recommended for the particular hairpiece.
- *Real* hair postiche must *not* be cleaned with shampoo or rinsed with water – this might result in tangling and loosening of the hair, and could shrink and distort the foundation base.

Cleaning synthetic fibre postiche

1 Add shampoo to a bowl of tepid water.
2 Gently move the postiche in the foamy water.
3 Rinse it in cool, clean water.

4 Repeat steps 1–3 if the postiche is still dirty. Rinse clear at the end.

5 The hairpiece may now be styled. Remember that too much brushing or combing can loosen the fibres.

Follow instructions when using other, recommended cleaners.

Cleaning real hair postiche

1 Do not use shampoo and water. Use recommended cleaners only and follow the instructions for their use. Use the cleaners in well-ventilated rooms – the fumes may be irritating.

2 Comb the postiche carefully before cleaning it.

3 Pour the cleaner into a bowl. Place the postiche in the cleaner, ensuring that the hair is covered.

4 Gently move the hairpiece in the cleaner for a minute or two; then lift it out and allow it to drain from the roots to the points.

5 Repeat steps 3 and 4 if necessary.

6 Remove any excess liquid, gently shaking the hairpiece, and allow the remaining liquid to evaporate, preferably in the open air.

7 When dry, styling may be carried out. If using water or setting lotions, keep these away from the foundation so as not to damage it.

An unclean piece of postiche can be irritating to wear. Be sure to clean it regularly.

HAIR EXTENSIONS

Hair extensions are lengths of processed hair or synthetic fibre (Monofibre™) similar in size and texture to hair in good condition. Clients whose hair is extended in this way have their 'hair' styled and shaped after the fibres have been attached. Styling may incorporate cutting, curling or dressing to achieve the desired effect.

Hair extensions bought from suppliers arrive in pre-packed, dyed, uniform lengths. Monofibre™ extensions are sold in packaged bundles called bales, whereas processed hair extensions arrive prepared and ready to apply.

Monofibre™ extensions are attached to the hair by a 'soldering' process which may last up to six months; processed hair extensions are attached much more frequently. The durability and condition of the extensions depend on many factors:

- the type of style
- the amount of extension hair
- the aftercare style maintenance
- the products used
- the styling equipment used.

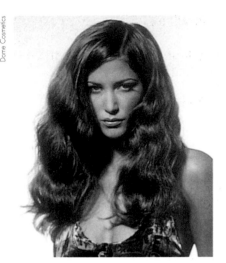

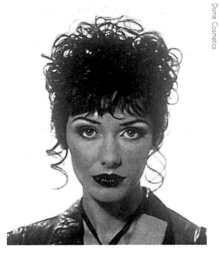

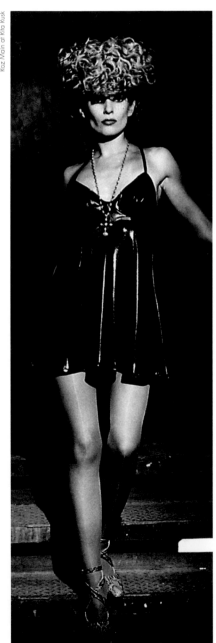

Bearing these controlling factors in mind, the style options for clients are limitless. Clients can have their hair lengthened, thickened, coloured or curled, all in one process.

The attachment of hair extensions to natural hair may involve the continuous assistance of other salon staff. During consultation with the client, this should be noted: the stylist should be able to estimate accurately how long it will take so that costings can remain profitable.

Synthetic fibre (Monofibre™) extensions

Apart from the traditional straight, waved or curled styling effects for clients, Monofibre™ extensions can be styled into dreadlocks, spindlelocks, bobtails, balls, cable curls, decorative braids or chaining. These effects are in addition to simply adding the hair, and can be made permanent by first twisting, backcombing or plaiting the hair to the required style, and then heating the applied fibre to fix its new structure permanently.

Special products are available for the aftercare of extensions, for cleaning, conditioning, fixing, gelling and waxing the fibre.

Although the bales of extensions bought are fairly limited in stock colours, unlike manufacturers' ranges of tints, different colours of fibre can be blended to produce a colour range far greater than any manufacturer's para-dye (permanent tint) spectrum. By blending different fibres it is possible to achieve highlights, lowlights, partial colour effects, varied colour effects and all-over colour effects.

Before a Monofibre™ hair-extension service can be provided, the stylist needs to know:

- what style is to be achieved
- what colour effect is to be achieved
- how long this will take
- how much fibre will be required
- who will be available if necessary to assist.

The client in turn will need to know:

- an accurate forecast of the cost
- what aftercare maintenance will be required
- the differences between handling hair and handling synthetic fibre
- how long the added hair may be expected to last.

After determining the style and colour (or colours) to be achieved, the first step is to select the appropriate tools and materials. Combs, brushes, clips, a heat-sealing device, bonding solution, styling sprays and the fibre itself should all be prepared before beginning the service.

HEALTH AND SAFETY

Synthetic hair extensions use a material similar to acrylic, which is quite unlike hair. If heated and bent, the fibres will remain permanently bent. Excessive heat will melt the extensions and may in turn burn the client's own hair and the scalp.

Clients should be made aware of the special care required in looking after hair extensions.

Colour principles for synthetic fibre extensions

Consider the mixing of paints. If you were to mix together 10 ml of black and 10 ml of white paint, you would expect to get 20 ml of grey paint. In the same way:

1 red (a) + white (b) → pink (c)
2 pink (c) + orange (d) → coral (e)
3 coral (e) + light brown (f) → chestnut (g)
4 chestnut (g) + yellow (h) → golden blonde (i)
5 golden blonde (i) + red (j) → vibrant copper (k).

By mixing a quantity of (a) with a quantity of (b), you achieve a different colour (c). This larger quantity of (c) can be mixed with a quantity of (d) to give (e), and so on.

Similarly, by mixing together two fibres you create a larger quantity of a third colour. With tints, the final, all-over colour effect is not seen until the hair has dried; with coloured fibres, however, the colour permutations are created immediately.

Megamixing is the process of mixing a number of colours together until the fibres are totally blended.

1 Decide on the colour or colours to be achieved.
2 Select the appropriate fibres to be mixed. Carefully remove the required amounts of fibre from the packs.
3 Take the base colour – the greatest amount – and place the fibres in the palm of your hand, holding them near one end. Place any secondary colours – the lesser amounts – on top. Close your fingers and hold the fibres tightly in your hand.

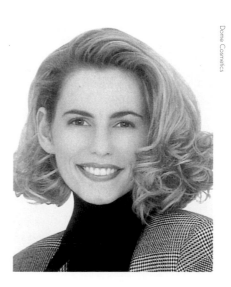

4 With your thumb, fan out the fibre along your first finger.

5 Now, using a bristle brush, brush the fibre downwards: this will tend to mix the fibres.

6 Hold the *opposite* end of the fibres in your palm and repeat this process: this will mix the fibres further.

7 Continue brushing and changing ends until the colours have been totally blended and the final colour is uniform.

Block colour gives a more defined colour or highlighting effect.

1 Take the base colour – the greater amount – and hold it centrally in the palm.

2 Lay the secondary colour – the lesser amount – on top, keeping the ends together.

3 Starting with your hands about 20 cm apart, bring your hands together. Divide the fibre into two equal amounts and separate your hands. Slight mixing will have occurred.

4 Again, place the fibre in one hand on top of the fibre in the other. The fibre is now all in one hand, partially mixed.

5 Bring your hands together and again divide the fibres into two. Further mixing will have occurred, but the fibres will still be in blocks of colour.

6 Repeat until the colour is sufficiently mixed.

7 *Gently* brush the fibre to remove any tangles, but not so as to mix the fibres further.

Attaching synthetic fibre extensions

1 Prepare the fibre to be used.

2 Prepare the heat-sealing device – clean it, select the temperature setting, and plug into the power point.

3 Prepare other tools and materials: combs, clips, brushes, scissors, styling sprays, and bonding solution (if required).

4 For hair extensions over the whole head, section the head into five areas.

5 Leave a 7 mm section of natural hair out around the hairline.

6 Start at the nape area. Take a band of hair above the hairline; secure the remainder out of the way with clips.

7 Starting in the centre of this band, take a section of hair 5 mm by 5 mm and again clip the remainder out of the way.

8 Divide the section of natural hair into two.

9 Your assistant now takes a similar amount of fibre and lays it centrally in between, forming a cross.

10 Cross the two pieces of natural hair over, right over left, and hold the hair apart while your assistant crosses left over right.

11 Cross again, right over left.

12 Your assistant leaves the top weft of fibre out and subdivides the bottom weft into two, pulling these apart so that you can cross over between them.

13 You both continue crossing until you have 12 mm of braided 'hair'.

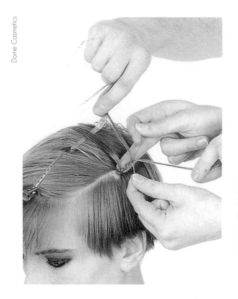
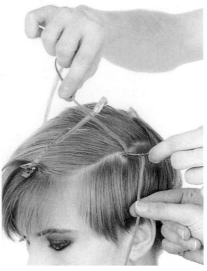

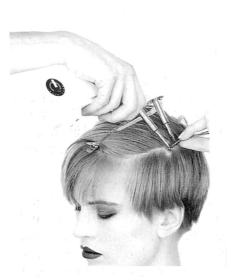
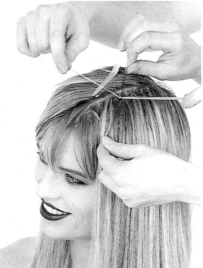

14 With your assistant holding the top of the plait between thumb and index finger, wrap the weft of fibre left out (step 12) around the braid.

15 With the heat sealer, close the tips over the bound braid approximately 20 mm down the braid. To close the tips, gently press them on to the fibre for 2 seconds. Lift the top tip and give a half turn, then close the tips again. Remove the heat after 2 seconds.

16 Pinch and roll the heated area between your fingers. Ensure that you have a smooth, round seal.

17 Repeat steps 1–16.

18 When the nape row is complete, continue up the head row by row.

19 After all the extensions have been applied, cut and dress the hair into the desired style.

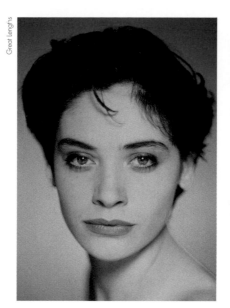
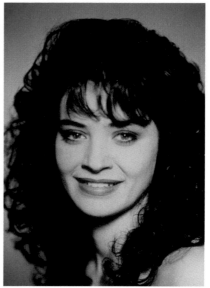

Processed (natural) hair extensions

Natural hair extensions provide alternative styling options to Monofibre™. Generally, styles created using Monofibre™ fall into the category of contemporary fashion effects, whereas the effects created by natural hair extensions are more traditional in their appearance. Routine hair management following the application of natural extensions is similar to working with human hair.

Natural hair extensions bought from the supplier arrive prepared by the manufacturer. They are available in a variety of strand colours, sizes and types – finer strands are for use around hairlines and partings, thicker strands are for use in other areas. You can also choose between straight, wavy and curly hair types. The wefts of hair are 'gummed' together with a polymer resin, so no colour blending is required – they are ready to attach to the hair.

Although the procedures for natural hair extensions may seem similar to those for synthetic hair extensions, in reality the processes are quite different. The polymer resin is activated by a device which emits ultra-high-frequency sound waves: once activated it moulds around the section of hair and creates a strong permanent bond.

Natural hair extensions can be styled by blow drying, tonging or using heated rollers. It is possible to use semi-permanent or temporary colours, but perming and tinting are not recommended.

Attaching processed hair extensions

1 Prepare the high-frequency equipment according to the manufacturer's instructions.
2 Prepare the other tools – the plastic strand shield, brushes, combs and clips, and whatever else you will need.

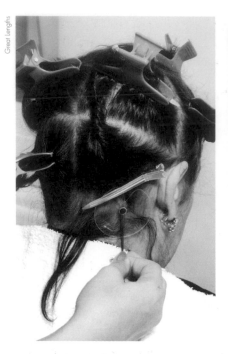

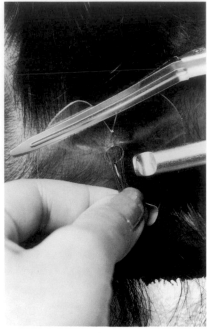

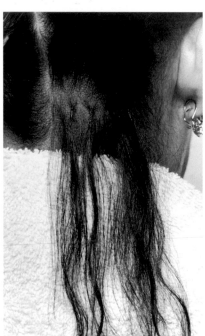

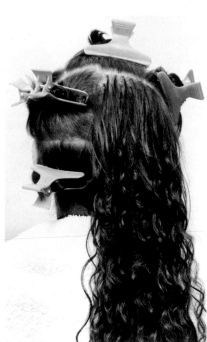

3 For hair extensions over the whole head, section the head
   into five working areas.
4 Leave a 7 mm section of hair out around the hairline.
5 Start at the nape area. Take a band of hair above the hairline;
   secure the remainder out of the way with clips.
6 Starting in the centre of this band, take a section of hair 5 mm
   by 5 mm and again clip the remainder out of the way.
7 Slide on the plastic protection shield and push it near to the
   scalp area.
8 Place the polymer-bonded end of the extension into the
   centre of the hair section, approximately 12 mm from the

scalp and forming a V-shaped wedge of hair around the bond. An even distribution of natural hair should surround the bonded end of the hair extension, to prevent uneven tension or breakage.

9 Place the grooved tip of the high-frequency device below the hair section.

10 Wait for the polymer to bubble before rolling it smoothly between your index finger and thumb. (Bubbling will occur in just a few seconds.)

11 Check that the bottom end of the bond is adequately sealed.

12 Continue the process, repeating steps 1–11 until the complete row is finished.

13 Continue working up the back of the head until the section is complete.

14 After all the extensions have been applied, cut and dress the hair into the desired style.

ORNAMENTATION AND HAIR ACCESSORIES

You can use a variety of ornaments or accessories as alternatives to added hairpieces to enhance your dressings. Combs, ribbons, bows, clasps, feathers, jewels, grips, slides, beads, sequins, flowers (real or artificial), glitterdust, coloured gels, coloured sprays, mousse, headbands, tiaras . . . all may be attractively used. Be discreet, however, in what you choose: a good dressing can be spoilt if the ornamentation is overdone.

Added colour is a popular means of augmenting shape and line throughout a dressing. Refer to Chapter 6 for more information on hair colouring.

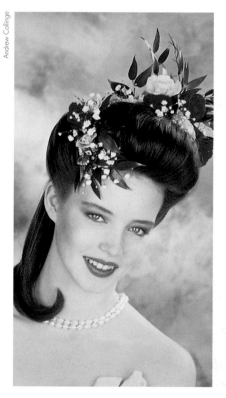

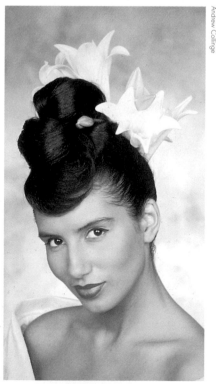

Special occasions

A special date, an interview for a new job, a party, or some other important event may be the occasion for a new hairstyle. Beware of changing just for the sake of it. Consider what is normally worn – the style may be suitable as it is and appropriate to the occasion.

Weddings and modelling or photographic sessions are important occasions. Hair styling for a wedding must take account of the headdress or tiara to be worn, as well as the dress and other accessories. Whatever is to be worn should be seen before hair styling is begun. Two or three dress rehearsals may be needed to ensure that all will be right on the day. Hair ornamentation, like the hairstyle, must complement the clothes to be worn: it must not 'intrude' on the ensemble.

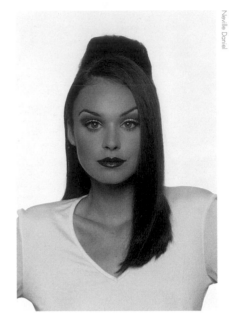

FASHION SETTING TECHNIQUES

Every day, hairdressers are faced with opportunities to make spontaneous and imaginative decisions. A client arrives and, after consultation and examination, a suitable course of action is agreed. A process then begins as the stylist attempts to achieve the desired result.

Hairdressers have never been restricted to using a set range of tools and equipment; new products arrive all the time. In order to achieve particular effects, hairdressers with flair, creativity and imagination have adapted or improvised with innumerable materials as they have sought to produce original and attractive

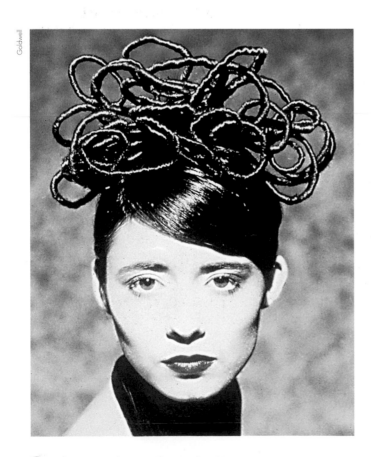

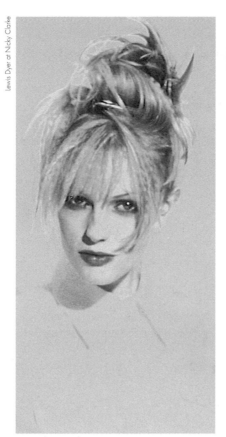

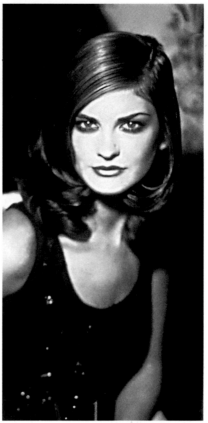

styles for their clients. This section could contain so much information that it would constitute a book by itself – a book that would be out of date before printing. As fashion moves on, therefore, remember only the *principles* of setting and dressing. Use your growing knowledge and skills to apply these principles creatively to achieve a variety of special, unusual effects. Consider the following:

- *Forming instruments* – the materials used to fix hair into place, including rubber or foam rollers; crimpers; U-stick rods, chopsticks, and spiral rods (see 'Alternative perming techniques' on page 86); Moulton Browners™ and spiral formers (which can also be used for perming).
- *Instrument positioning* – the techniques of applying the instrument to the hair.
- *Dressing requirements* – the styling and dressing needed to achieve the desired effect, as with sculptured fashion styles.
- *Styling aids* – the plethora of sprays, lotions, mousses, gels, creams and waxes now available to the hairdresser.

ASSIGNMENT

With the permission of your manager, carry out a work-based assignment in which you produce materials for use in your portfolio.

For this assignment, you will need to provide sketches and/or photographs with explanatory notes for the following dressing procedures:

- upswept knots and rolls
- plaiting, twisting and weaving
- added hair and hairpieces
- ornamentation
- fashion setting techniques.

After carrying out each of the practical tasks listed above, write explanatory illustrated notes to show:

1 how the effects were achieved

2 the variety of tools, equipment and products used

3 a range of hairpieces and hair ornaments, stating how they were attached and where they can be obtained

4 the relevant health, safety and hygiene requirements.

You may prefer not to compile sketches, photographs and accompanying notes, but instead to video the entire practical tasks and then to give a personal account of what has taken place. Make sure that you address points 1–4 within your account.

QUESTIONS

After completing the assignment, answer these questions in your portfolio.

1 What are the differences between knots, plaits, pleats and weaves?

2 Name the different types of postiche available for ornamentation. How would you use each of them?

3 List the various means of ornamentation. Describe how and when you would use them.

4 How would you arrive at a 'suitable' dressing for your client? List the points to be considered.

5 Describe the effects produced by the various setting and drying techniques.

CHAPTER 8

African-Caribbean hair techniques

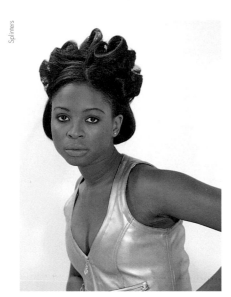

Splinters

INTRODUCTION

In this chapter we will look at working with African-Caribbean hair and providing related services. These techniques are not exclusively for the African-Caribbean client, but can also be used to style multi-textured hair.

The specialist elements to African-Caribbean hairdressing are:

- using heated equipment to style hair
- relaxing hair.

Some of the most experienced hairdressers fear this kind of work: it is an area which needs to be understood and practised like any other technical specialism, for example colouring or perming. With product knowledge, technical knowledge and the development of practical skill, African-Caribbean techniques can be mastered.

CONSULTATION

The stylist should go through the following points mentally, and in consultation with the client, to determine procedure:

- *The client and her lifestyle* See Chapter 3 for more information on the relevance of this in deciding on the correct procedure.
- *The ethnic origins of the client to assist hair type analysis* Information about the client's ethnic origins will help you work out exactly what chemical or heat treatments to use, and in what strengths.
- *Hair and scalp condition* Is the client's hair virgin or treated? Is the texture curly, wavy or straight? If curly, note the pattern, type and circumference of the curls. What is the hair's present porosity level? The moisture or porosity level of the hair is highly important when working with the African-Caribbean hair type, as the chemical and styling processes used deplete the moisture level rapidly. This can lead to irrevocable damage unless monitored carefully.
- *Date and type of the client's last treatment* If the hair has been treated, ascertain exactly what has been done to it in the past and how long ago this was carried out.
- *The desired final effect* What kind of style does the client want you to create? Is this going to be possible, taking the above factors into consideration?

STYLING HAIR USING HEATED EQUIPMENT

Preparing the client

Preparing the tools and equipment

Preparing the oven

Danger areas

Sectioning the hair

Preparing the client

- [ ] Cleanse the hair, selecting and using the right shampoo.
- [ ] Condition the hair. *Always* use a conditioner with a moisture humectant. Make use of the leave-in conditioners as well.
- [ ] Dry the hair. Select the appropriate method of drying the hair. Even tension is important. To make sure you get an even result, the hair needs to be straight before being pressed or tonged. Hair can be blown out using the comb attachment on the dryer, or set in rollers.
- [ ] Heated styling is not recommended when the hair has been curly permed. If it is done on occasion, the hair should be roller set, not blown out.

Preparing the tools and equipment

Are you going to press or tong the hair?
Collect together the equipment you will need.

Pressing is a soft method, where the perimeter surface of the hair shaft is straightened using a steel comb. It is used either when a soft press is required due to the levels of porosity and elasticity, or for regrowth straightening between relaxers. It is an ideal way of straightening hairline areas close to the scalp.

Tonging is a hard method, using tongs which clamp both sides of the hair section, transferring more heat to the section and creating a straighter, longer-lasting finish. It is used to create a number of styles, with the selection of tong circumference determining the final result.

To heat style hair, you will need:

- a hairdryer with a comb attachment
- a Denman D4 hairbrush, or similar
- a tailcomb
- sectioning clips
- the oven
- a pressing comb and a selection of tongs
- thermal spray and/or oil spray
- setting agents.

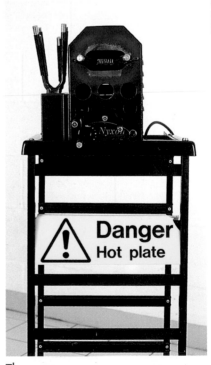

Ian Flanders

The oven

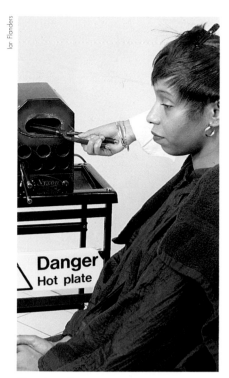

Heating the tongs

Preparing the oven

☐ Make sure the tongs and combs are suitable for the oven.
☐ Heat test the tongs with a piece of paper to make sure they are not too hot.

The oven is a specialist piece of equipment. It is electrically operated, and heats to a temperature of 70°C. The combs and tongs available for use in the oven must be recommended and approved by the manufacturer. Health and safety rules state that a yellow warning plaque should be displayed by the oven.

Once the oven is ready for use, the comb or tong is placed inside for 5–20 seconds. Before placing the tong on to the hair, it must be temperature tested. This is done by sliding the tong on to a white end paper. If it singes or scorches the paper, do *not* place it on the hair.

Working with heated equipment requires skill and practice. Extreme heat damages hair. It is therefore always necessary to coat the hair with a thermal styling lotion before the heated equipment touches the hair.

Danger areas

☐ If you burn the hair, it will break off.
☐ Take care, especially around the ears and hairline, so you do not burn your client's skin.
☐ Watch the hair colour: if lightening occurs, apply semi-permanent conditioning.

Do you know the salon procedure for dealing with client complaints? Who is responsible for first aid and health and safety in the salon?

Sectioning the hair

☐ Follow the nine section or directional perming pattern.
☐ Always start at the nape and work forward, with the front hairline the last section.
☐ Ensure your client is satisfied and that the style of work reflects the salon image.
☐ Oil sheens may be used following heat. Advise the client of the correct home care and recommend appropriate products.

Tonging the hair – start at the nape and work forward

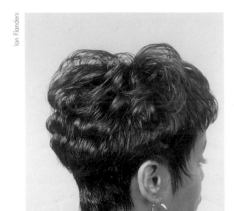

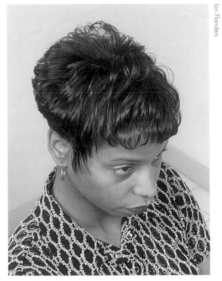

Tonging – the finished effect

ROUTINE AND CORRECTIVE HAIR RELAXING SERVICES

Product knowledge

Preparing for the treatment

Application

Aftercare

Product knowledge

- Hair relaxers are among the most dangerous chemical treatments in the salon.
- Thorough client consultation is essential.

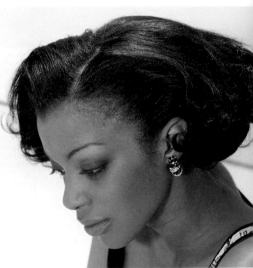

Ian Flanders

Sodium hydroxide based relaxers

These are available in three strengths: super, regular and mild. They are professional products, recommended for salon use only. They have a rapid development time, and continue working until they are removed and neutralised. They are extremely alkaline, having a pH of 10–14. They are the most effective way of chemically straightening hair.

Calcium based 'no-lye' relaxers

These are available in two strengths: sensitive and mild. They are marketed and sold as home treatment products. They are slower acting, with a pH of 7.5–8, and they have a longer development time.

> **HEALTH AND SAFETY**
> Sodium hydroxide can burn the skin and scalp, make the hair brittle and break, and dissolve the hair. *Always* follow the manufacturer's instructions.

> **HEALTH AND SAFETY**
> Prolonged development time makes the hair brittle and lacking in moisture.

Preparing for the treatment

☐ Refer to the record card for past treatments.
☐ If the client is new to the salon, begin with an incompatibility strand test.
☐ Consider the hair type and the sensitivity of the scalp.

When you are checking the record card, remember that the client may have had other treatments between salon visits, which should be identified.

Carry out the strand test by applying selected relaxer to a few strands of hair. Check the elasticity level and select the appropriate relaxing product. Take into account the texture, porosity and elasticity of the hair, and the sensitivity of the scalp. The most accurate way of doing this is to apply some product directly on to a small area of scalp, having first checked for cuts and abrasions.

Hair types vary from fine and porous through to coarse and resistant. It is quite possible to have the combination of resistant hair with a sensitive scalp.

Application

☐ The whole process, from basing the scalp to removing the relaxer, should take no more than 30 minutes. Speed is essential.
☐ Relaxers are applied to dry hair.
☐ To minimise scalp discomfort, the hair should not be shampooed for at least three days.
☐ Basing the scalp is essential and should be done with great care. Working through the traditional hot cross bun method, small horizontal sections are taken from the nape forward to the front hairline. A thin layer of petroleum jelly is applied to the scalp. This prevents product contact with the scalp. The base application should be extended around the ears, the forehead and the neck.

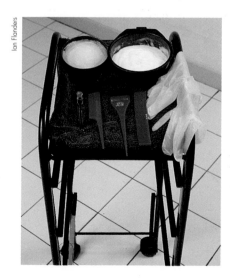

Ian Flanders

Virgin application

1 Section the hair into four, like a hot cross bun.
2 Starting at the nape, take horizontal sections and apply the product directly with the hands to the mid-lengths and ends.
3 Work through until the hair begins to soften, then apply to the root area. The product should be a millimetre from the scalp.

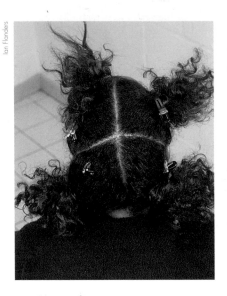
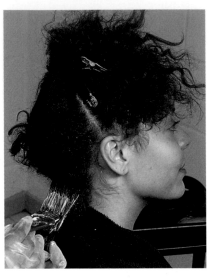

Virgin application

Regrowth application

1 Divide the hair into four sections as before.
2 Lay a small amount of product on to the hair, working from the nape forward to the front hairline.
3 Once the application is completed, return to the nape area and, following the same sections, gently comb through, using a fine-tooth comb and maintaining even tension.

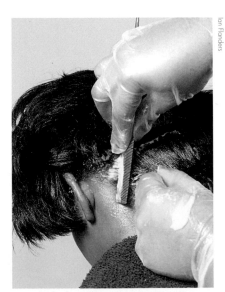

Comb the product through with a fine-tooth comb

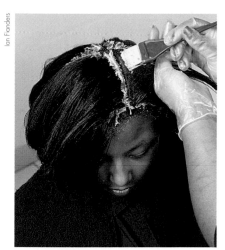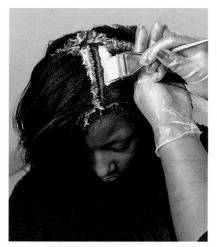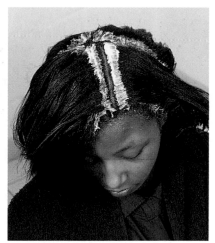

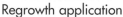
Regrowth application

HEALTH AND SAFETY
Never use a sodium hydroxide or calcium hydroxide base to straighten thioglycolate processed hair – that is, *never straighten permed hair with relaxer.*

Texturising and partial relaxing

Texturising is suitable for naturally curly hair to reduce the tightness and appearance of curl, and for fine hair.

1 Working through the same sectioning pattern, use one application only and comb through gently with a wide-spaced tooth comb.
2 Develop for 5–10 minutes, then rinse, shampoo and condition.

Corrective relaxing

This will be necessary when there has been an uneven application during prior treatments.

1 The hair must be wet for analysing.
2 Section through to see which areas need processing.
3 Dry the hair in its natural state – that is, under the heat lamps – and follow the application procedure.

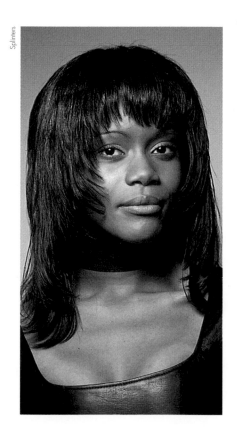

HEALTH AND SAFETY
Always remember the following points when working with chemicals:
• wear protective gloves
• cover clothes with an apron
• ensure the client is correctly gowned, with clean towels around the neck; disposable capes may be used to protect the towels.

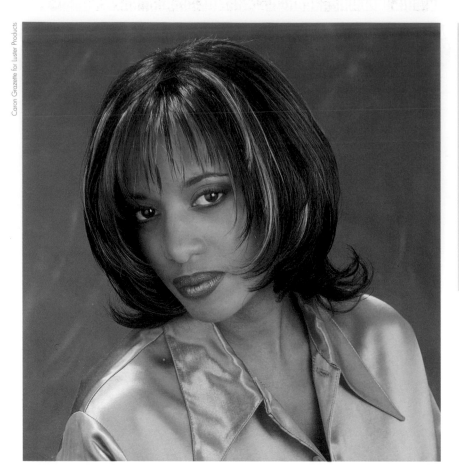

Caron Grazette for Luster Products

Client aftercare

- Recommend regular steam treatments of protein and moisture to keep the hair in the best possible condition for ongoing chemical treatments and heated styling.
- Recommend suitable shampoos, conditioners, deep conditioning treatments and oils for the client to use between salon visits.

ASSIGNMENT

With the permission of your manager, carry out a work-based assignment in which you produce materials for use in your portfolio.

For this assignment, you will need to provide sketches and/or photographs with explanatory notes for the following processes:

- basing the scalp in preparation for chemical relaxation
- applying a relaxer to a regrowth of previously treated hairs
- a partial application for corrective purposes
- styling hair using tongs (from the oven).

After carrying out each of the practical tasks listed above, write explanatory illustrated notes to show:

1 how the final effects were achieved
2 the selection of tools, equipment and products used
3 the effects and potential effects of using chemical relaxers on virgin and previously treated hair
4 the potential problems which might have occurred and what remedial action is appropriate in each case
5 the relevant health, safety and hygiene requirements.

You may prefer not to compile sketches, photographs and accompanying notes, but instead to video the entire practical tasks and then to give a personal account of what has taken place. Make sure that you address points 1–5 within your account.

QUESTIONS

After completing the assignment, answer these questions in your portfolio.

1 Describe the process of applying a chemical relaxer to (a) a regrowth area, and (b) virgin hair.
2 List the main points of a client consultation prior to conducting a chemical service.
3 What aftercare is recommended for clients who have chemical or heated styling treatments?
4 What length of time should be allowed between treatments?

150 PROFESSIONAL HAIRDRESSING

CHAPTER 9

Working as a team

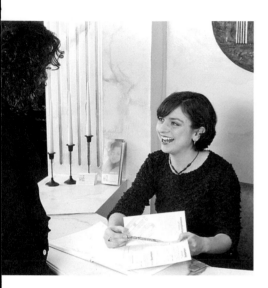

INTRODUCTION

This chapter is about working together productively as a team and covers the following topics:

- getting yourself organised
- effective communication
- how to work as part of a team
- personal development.
- discipline and grievance procedures.

It also looks in detail at the role of the supervisor, including:

- planning staff cover
- allocating work
- supporting staff.

GETTING ORGANISED

All salons use the same tabular system for organising work, although different salons use this system in differing ways. The appointment system provides them with the following:

- a daily detailed action plan
- a schedule of individual work allocations
- a clear overview of business activities
- a general indication of expected time scales
- a general indication of expected sales.

The appointment system also has direct links with:

- resource requirements (such as stock and equipment)
- client records
- till transactions (such as daily sheets and till rolls).

As you can see, this system is the hub of an efficiently run business. The information it contains must therefore be clear, accurate and up to date.

But maintaining the appointment system correctly will not ensure the smooth running of the salon. You will always need to be prepared for the unexpected!

Your salon may have specific contingency procedures for coping with the following unplanned situations and circumstances, but generally the simple rules described here apply.

Late arrivals of clients

Suppose that a client arrives 15 minutes late for her appointment and apologetically explains that she was unavoidably held up (in circumstances beyond her control). What should you do?

First and foremost, be sympathetic and understanding. Find out if her stylist has still sufficient time to provide the service. If not, find out if anyone else can attend to her needs. Find out how long she may have to wait (if at all). Will there be any extra costs to the client? Will the appointment have to be rebooked?

Arrivals of unscheduled clients

A client who arrives unexpectedly without a booked appointment should always be accommodated, provided that there is an operator available and sufficient time to carry out the service or treatment.

Overbooking

This does occur but, it is to be hoped, not too often. Normally this situation arises accidentally when a client or a staff member has made a mistake, or through poor communications. Deliberate overbooking is only done by over-optimistic staff members. The result is that other people will need to be drawn in to help; otherwise delays will be unavoidable.

Don't try to beat the appointment system; you may upset clients, colleagues or both. Providing a high-quality service includes making sure people know the expected time scales and duration of services and treatments, and if there will be any waiting.

Changes to booked requirements

It often happens that a client who has booked for one service will, following consultation, change her mind and require something different. Don't worry! This could be good business – a client may come in expecting a restyle cut and finish, and go out with a change of hair colour as well. In fact many salons set incentives around this type of situation; for example, staff performances and/or commissions may be based on numbers of 'customer conversions'.

Staff absences

Staff absence will always stretch the salon to its limits, but your salon should have contingency plans to cover this situation. Generally this will involve:

- checking customer records to see if other staff members have provided the service previously
- checking availability of appointments with other staff at the same time

- rescheduling in the appropriate spaces
- if all else fails, contacting the client to rebook the appointment at a later date.

EFFECTIVE COMMUNICATION

Good communication is always important – not just between clients and staff, but also between staff and management.

Most hairdressers are good communicators. The relationship between stylist and client is built on quality of service, professional advice, trust, support and a listening ear.

Good communication ensures productive and effective action and promotes the ongoing success of the business. On the other hand poor communication, arising from misunderstanding or misinterpretation, can lead to mistrust, arguments and embarrassment.

Written communication

A *memorandum* (or *memo*) is an ideal means of providing a written communication to team members. An effective memo clearly indicates:

- to whom it is addressed
- who wrote it
- the date
- the purpose of the memo
- its content (including, if relevant, clear and concise instructions).

Keep copies of your memos so that you and individual staff members have a record.

Memorandum

TO: John
FROM: Linda
DATE: 1/10
SUBJECT: Staff Absence

Jayne will not be in for the rest of the week. Please could you reschedule her appointments, and advise all clients accordingly.
Thanks.

Oral communication

When providing information to others, whether face to face or on the telephone, remember to speak clearly; don't waffle, and try not to speak too fast. Be polite and listen carefully to the other's responses. To check that the information has been received correctly, ask if you have been understood and heard clearly. If not, repeat the main content of the information.

Body language

As well as using words, we express our interest and attitudes by non-verbal communication – our eye contact, posture and general body positioning. So it is very important that we convey the right *message*, particularly when dealing with clients and potential customers.

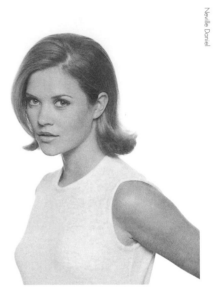

Eye contact

Maintain eye contact with the client when talking to her. Where possible, maintain the same eye level as the client; for example, when you carry out a consultation with a client and she is seated, sit beside or opposite her. Standing over or above her and looking down will convey a feeling of authority, and might appear as if you are trying to assert control. This is intimidating and definitely the wrong signal to send to a customer.

Distance

People have a 'comfort zone', a space around the body within which they feel at ease. Within a close, intimate relationship, shared proximity may be welcome, but uninvited invasion of this space is at least uncomfortable, at worst menacing or threatening.

Posture/body positioning/gestures

Volumes have been written on this subject alone and the psychology of body language is far too complex to address in a few paragraphs. But following certain obvious 'rules' can help us convey the right message and impression.

- Slouching in the salon looks very unprofessional.
- Folded arms – crossing the arms on the chest is a protective gesture and suggests a closed mind or a show of defensiveness.
- Open palms – as a gesture supporting explanation or information, with hands at waist height, palms upwards, this indicates that the person has 'nothing to hide'. This is interpreted as openness or honesty.
- Scratching behind the ear or rubbing the back of the neck while listening indicates that the listener is uncertain or doesn't understand.

- Talking with your hand in front of your mouth may lead the listener to believe that you are not being honest. You are hiding yourself by your gestures.

These forms of communication are only indications of feelings and emotions. In isolation, they may not mean anything at all. Taken together, however, they can convey a very clear message. Make sure that you show the appropriate signals; be – and look – interested, keen, ready to help and positive. Above all, show that you can listen.

Meetings

Formal and informal meetings provide opportunities for gathering and passing on information and advice. Regular team meetings allow individuals to voice opinions and suggestions – these don't always come to light in day-to-day interactions.

Informal meetings

Informal (unplanned) meetings can be useful, but unless the information or recommendations that come out of them are recorded in some way, they may get forgotten.

Formal meetings

Formal (planned) meetings are basic to communication with companies throughout the commercial world. They are a device for channelling information to and from management. Successful meetings need careful planning:

- Identify the purpose of the meeting.
- Provide a written *agenda,* indicating all the topics for consideration.
- Send invitations to those who will be asked to contribute or who may benefit in some respect from attending.
- Ensure comfortable facilities, appropriate to the needs of the meeting.
- Check that resources are available as necessary to be used in presenting information.
- Afterwards, compile a summary or minutes which can be distributed to all who attended the meeting.

WORKING AS A TEAM

Always remember that your work colleagues need your assistance to help them do their job. Sharing the workload *is* working as a team. This can be achieved by:

- providing support
- anticipating the needs of others
- maintaining harmony
- maintaining good communication.

In some salons, you might see some staff busy attending to their clients, but others hanging about around reception, flicking through magazines or disappearing off to the staff room for a coffee. Teamwork is about making an active contribution, seeking to assist others even if it is only passing up rollers. It is good for staff morale and presents a good image to the clients. In short, make yourself useful and contribute to the team effort by assisting your fellow workers.

Anticipating the needs of others follows on from providing support. Clean and prepare the work areas ready for use, locate and prepare products as and when they are required. (This will help the smooth operation of the salon.) Cooperate with your colleagues – make a positive contribution to your team by assisting them to provide a well-managed and coordinated quality service. Be self-motivated; keep yourself busy. Don't wait to be asked to do things.

Maintain harmony and try to minimise possible conflicts. Most good working relationships develop easily; others, however, need to be worked at.

Whatever your personal feelings are about your fellow work associates, clients must never sense a bad atmosphere within the salon caused by a friction between staff. You will spend a lot of time in the company of people you work with, but you will not always like everyone you meet. People are different: at work, in order to work as a team, a mutual respect for others is more important than close friendships. So remember:

- treat others with respect
- be sensitive and responsive to others' feelings
- show concern and care for others.

PERSONAL DEVELOPMENT

Managers of people use *performance appraisal* or *progress reviews* to evaluate the effectiveness of the work team. An appraisal is a system whereby you and your manager, in an interview situation, review and evaluate your personal contribution and/or progress over a predetermined period of time, as measured against expected targets or standards.

A similar process would take place at suitable points within a personal programme of training in order to review progress and training effectiveness, measured against specific training objectives.

An appraisal form

Performance Appraisal

Name:	*Jane Manners*
Job Title:	*Trainee stylist*
Date of Appraisal:	*30/10/97*
Objectives:	*To obtain competence within:-* *Cutting hair – layering techniques across the range.* *Blow drying hair – on a variety of hair types* *and lengths*
Notes on Achievement:	*- competence has been achieved across the range* *for all the cutting requirements.* *- competence has been achieved for most blow* *drying range requirements*
Training Requirements:	*Further training and practice is needed within the* *area of blow drying longer length effects.*
Any other comments on performance by Appraiser:	*Jane has achieved most of the objectives set out* *during the last appraisal.*
Any comments on the Appraisal by the staff Appraised:	*I feel that this has been a fair appraisal of my* *progress although I did not achieve all of my* *performance targets.* *Jane Manners*
Action Plan:	*- To achieve occupational competence across the* *range for blow drying (i.e. longer length hair).* *- To undergo training and practice in perming* *methods and techniques.* *- To take assessment for perming.*
Date of Next Appraisal:	*28 April 1998*

Measuring effectiveness

To measure progress towards training targets as well as overall work contributions, there needs to be clear stated expectations of the performance required. For both training and work activities, this is the standard in which competence will need to be demonstrated.

In training situations, trainees undergo a programme of training which states:

- what training activities will take place
- what tasks need to be performed
- what standards are expected to be reached
- when assessment should be expected
- when a review of progress towards the agreed targets is to take place.

In normal, ongoing work situations, performance appraisal will be based on the following factors:

- results achieved against objectives and job requirements
- any additional accomplishments and contributions
- contributions made by the individual as compared with those of other staff members.

The job requirements would be outlined in the employee's *job description*. A job description is a written specification of the main purposes and functions expected within a given job. Good job descriptions will include details of the following:

- the job title
- the work location(s)

Job description – Stylist

Location:	Based at salon as advised
Main purpose of job:	To ensure customer care is provided at all times To maintain a good standard of technical and client care, ensuring that up-to-date methods and techniques are used following the salon training practices and procedures
Responsible to:	Salon manager
Requirements:	To maintain the company's standards in respect of hairdressing/beauty services
	To ensure that all clients receive service of the best possible quality
	To advise clients on services and treatments
	To advise clients on products and aftercare
	To achieve designated performance targets
	To participate in self-development or to assist with the development of others
	To maintain company policy in respect of: • personal standards of health/hygiene • personal standards of appearance/conduct • operating safety whilst at work • public promotion • corporate image as laid out in employee handbook
	To carry out client consultation in accordance with company policy
	To maintain company security practices and procedures
	To assist your manager in the provision of salon resources
	To undertake additional tasks and duties required by your manager from time to time.

- responsibility (to whom, and for what)
- the job purpose
- main functions (listed)
- standards expected
- any special conditions.

Standards expected from the job holder will often include standards of behaviour and appearance. If these have been stated from the outset, the job holder will know what is expected of her.

The appraisal process

At the beginning of the appraisal period, the manager and the employee discuss jointly, develop, and mutually agree the objectives and performance measures for that period. An *action plan* will then be drafted, outlining the expected outcomes.

During the appraisal period, should there be any significant changes in factors such as objectives or performance measures, these will be discussed between the manager and employee and any amendments will be appended to the action plan.

At the end of the appraisal period, the results are discussed by the employee and the manager, and both manager and employee sign the appraisal. A copy is prepared for the employee and the original is kept on file.

An appraisal of performance will contain the following information:

- employee's name
- appraisal period
- appraiser's name and title
- performance objectives
- job title
- work location
- results achieved
- identified areas of strength and weakness
- ongoing action plan
- overall performance grading (optional).

Self-appraisal

In order for you to manage yourself within the job role, you need to identify the areas where you meet the expectations of your job and also the areas where there is room for improvement. Measuring your own strengths and weaknesses against laid-down performance criteria (as found in the NVQ Level 3 standards of competence) is one way of monitoring your own progress. Simply use the performance criteria set out within the standards as a checklist; this will help you to:

- identify areas where further training is required
- identify areas where further practice is required
- identify areas where competence can be achieved.

Occupational Standard
Unit 4 Enhance the overall effectivenes of the work team

Element 4.2
Enhance personal effectiveness within the job role

Performance criteria

a) own strengths and weaknesses within the job role are identified with the immediate manager, taking into account organisational and national occupational standards, and relevant legislation
b) potential for improving effectiveness is identified with the immediate manager and realistic targets agreed
c) opportunities available for improving self-motivation and effectiveness are actively sought and are used to best effect
d) progress towards achievement of agreed targets is reviewed regularly with the immediate manager
e) results of reviews are used constructively to assist personal development
f) awareness of current and emerging fashion trends and developments in technology within the industry is maintained

Range statements

i) Developments in technology:
   • products and their usage
   • tools
   • equipment

Essential knowledge and understanding requirements

• How to identify own strengths and weaknesses
• How to react positively to reviews and feedback, and why this is important
• How to maintain awareness of current emerging trends and developments within the industry, and why this is important

NVQ standard

THE ROLE OF THE SUPERVISOR

Managers are the people who make decisions about the running of the business. Often they are administrators who lack the technical expertise to assess or evaluate the individual performances of stylists and trainees. It is the *supervisor*, therefore, who bridges the gap between strategic planning and shop-floor activities: she is the key link in communication.

The salon supervisor assists management in allocating work to staff. She also reports back to management on the effectiveness and efficiency of individual and team performances. She must therefore be able to analyse and evaluate working practices; when necessary she must make spontaneous decisions about staff cover in the event of abnormal working conditions. Systematic allocation of tasks and contingency planning by the supervisor ensure the smooth, efficient operation of the salon.

Supporting management

Strategic planning is the responsibility of the manager: it is your job, as supervisor, to support the manager in her decisions.

You are directly involved with the implementation of practices and procedures, and with your own technical expertise you should be able to monitor progress and evaluate the effectiveness of any plan. If systems are found to be unworkable, you can recommend alternative solutions or courses of action. In negotiating with your manager, give reasons for your suggestions.

Whenever you change a plan or system, the change has some effect on someone or something. You may be better placed than the manager to foresee the implications of a proposed change. Giving feedback based on informed opinion is supporting your manager in a positive way.

As supervisor you are expected to have a working knowledge of the legislation and the company policy affecting your working environment. Some recommendations for change, although sound in principle, cannot be put into practice because of legal constraints. Alternative solutions must then be sought.

Planning staff cover

The planning of staff cover will depend on your salon's resources. A small, independent salon with only a few staff members will often find it difficult to cover for absences, holidays and unexpected busy periods; this problem can occur with large companies too.

It is the supervisor's job, whatever the salon staffing level, to plan and maintain adequate cover in all circumstances. Provided that individuals are adequately trained and briefed, you should be able to manage this.

The first thing you should do is to evaluate the current levels of competence. This can be done by referring to staff records of:

- employment
- training and assessment
- staff appraisal.

With this information, provided that it has been kept up to date, you should be able to devise a system that records current experience and skill. These could be recorded under the following headings:

- technical/craft ability
- communication skills
- administrative skills.

The value of this becomes apparent if you imagine the problems that could occur if someone who was allocated to reception duties couldn't use the till, schedule appointments or handle telephone enquiries!

Contingency planning

If you have made the necessary preparations, providing cover for predictable disruptions such as tea breaks, lunch breaks and holidays shouldn't be a problem. What is difficult is planning for unusual circumstances arising from unexpected absences which stretch the salon resources to the limits. Consider the following scenario:

It is 8.30 on Saturday morning. The receptionist receives a telephone call from one of the stylists who reports that she is sick and will not be able to work today.

Looking at the appointment book, you see that this stylist was due to be very busy: first there is a wedding party (bride and maids); three clients are booked during the mid-morning and early afternoon for perms or colours; and the rest of the day is made up of regular clients having cutting or styling services.

You have to make decisions immediately. First, prioritise the work according to the customers' needs and the salon's goodwill. After considering the existing staff cover, you are left with two categories: services and treatments that will be provided, and services and treatments that must be deferred.

If you have given jobs priorities, you will probably be thinking along these lines:

1 Were any *other* staff involved with the selection of styles and effects during the wedding group's trial runs? If so, can they either carry out the service themselves or convey the client's wishes to another stylist?
2 Check customer records and evaluate the service and treatment history. Note any special conditions or relevant remarks, and the time scales involved for the planned services.
3 Reschedule as many customers as possible with appropriate members of staff.
4 Where rescheduling is not possible, arrange for the customers to be contacted so that new appointments may be made.
5 Brief all the staff members involved, explaining the amendments made to the original bookings.

	Saturday March 23rd
	JANICE
8.30	Stilby
8.45	BRIDE/PUT UP
9.00	JONES
9.15	B/D Bridesmaid
9.30	JONES
9.45	S/SET Bridesmaid
10.00	/////
10.15	
10.30	PORTMAN
10.45	Perm/Long hair
11.00	/////
11.15	JAMES
11.30	RETOUCH COLOUR
11.45	JAMES/dry cut
12.00	PERM/NAT DRY
12.15	

Appointment book extract

Allocating work

If you plan comprehensively to cover all the eventualities you can think of, you will have maximised the potential work output for all the salon personnel.

One fundamental problem facing salons nationwide is individual popularity and success. A hairdresser's popularity may be due to many factors, not all related to her hairdressing skills. It is your job as salon supervisor to distribute the workload evenly at any one time.

Companies cannot afford to 'carry' personnel who don't pull their weight, whether through lack of customer demand or because of individual laziness. It is your job to ensure that your staff work as a team. Hairdressing is a labour-intensive occupation, but clients see only the skills used in salon operations. The levels of support and maintenance required daily behind the scenes provide enough work for all spare hands, regardless of whether they belong to stylists, trainees, ancillary staff or those on work experience.

If you succeed in maintaining an even balance of work distribution, you will find that staff:

- remain happier in their work
- feel that their input is useful
- are less likely to cause disputes.

Supporting and supervising staff

The support given during training requires you to coach individuals while they learn. Supervisory support can be quite different from training support: you are concerned to measure the effectiveness and the efficiency of specific tasks being performed. Generally your level of support should take the form of casual observation, perhaps providing feedback later at a mutually convenient time. It is usually inappropriate to ask staff members in front of paying clients whether or not they can cope: that condescending style of management makes it hard to build good working relationships. You *must* tactfully intervene, however, whenever practices and procedures are not being carried out safely or satisfactorily, or where the individual:

- is not yet competent in a given activity
- lacks the necessary confidence
- needs further instruction.

Minimising conflict

In some salons the manager is not always available; she may in any case not be a practising hairdresser. In such an environment the supervisor plays a key role, in evaluating:

- individual staff performance
- staff attitudes
- the social wellbeing of the staff.

As a practising hairdresser yourself, it will be relatively easy for you to measure the competence of your team.

Problems with individuals

A particular member of staff may show evidence of an 'attitude problem'. In doing so she may upset other members of staff, or even your clients. It is essential that you select an appropriate time and a private place to discuss this with the individual, explaining the problem as you see it and listening to the other person's point of view. You must show a caring but firm attitude when dealing with disruptive behaviour: failure to do so may make the situation worse. In particular, if you don't listen as well as talk you may push this member of staff into being rebellious and uncooperative. Remember, any judgements you make should be based on facts and informed opinion, *not* supposition and rumour.

Information of a personal or private nature must always be handled with discretion. If your manager needs to be involved, offer your support and if necessary assist the individual at any interview with the manager.

Equal opportunities

In the past, staff in many organisations felt that they were at a disadvantage because of their sex, race or disability. Changing attitudes and the easing of European trade restrictions have improved this situation, but you need to be vigilant in preventing any discrimination.

Employment legislation now requires codes of practice and policy statements which address these issues: these should be provided by all companies. The following is an example of an equal opportunities statement, produced by the Department of Employment.

EQUAL OPPORTUNITIES STATEMENT

The company wholeheartedly supports the principle of equal opportunities in employment and opposes all forms of unlawful or unfair discrimination on the grounds of colour, race, nationality, ethnic or national origin, sex, being married or disability. We believe that it is in the company's best interests, and those of all who work in it, to ensure that the human resources, talents and skills available throughout the community are considered when employment opportunities arise. To this end, within the framework of the law, we are committed, wherever practicable, to achieving and maintaining a workforce which broadly reflects the local community in which we operate.

Every possible step will be taken to ensure that individuals are treated equally and fairly and that decisions on recruitment, selection, training, promotion, and career management are based solely on objective and job related criteria.

DISCIPLINARY ACTION

This book has continually referred to the standards of competence that the industry expects. Your company will have additional standards, relating to conduct and behaviour. Preventative action is better than cure, so staff will be happier in their work if they know what is expected of them. These rules and working conditions can be clarified and displayed through job descriptions and organisational policy.

Organisational policy

Within an organisation's policy there should be an outline of the required performance levels relating to each aspect of the business:

- health and safety procedures
- the security of company resources
- systems and documentation
- staff relationships
- customer care and company goodwill
- punctuality and absence
- dismissible offences (usually, forms of gross misconduct)
- grievance procedures.

The organisational policy should be displayed or individually copied to all concerned. Many companies produce a handbook or guide which is given to new staff members during their induction. This may contain policy statements as well as legal requirements.

Disciplinary action: a suggested procedure

If staff members fail to meet the required standards, they should expect disciplinary action to be taken against them.

It is wise to have a formal procedure for this, with known stages:

1 *Verbal warning* This should be witnessed, and the date and circumstances recorded in case it is necessary to refer to it later.
2 *Second verbal warning* Again, this should be witnessed and documented. Note that it must concern the same matter as the first warning.
3 *Final (written) warning* This must be given to the staff member in writing. It should refer to the previous verbal warnings. A final warning could result in dismissal, so only the manager can implement this action.
4 *Dismissal.*

If disciplinary action results in a third and final warning, the manager will conduct an interview with the employee in order to:

- establish the facts
- weigh the evidence
- decide the future course of action.

Supervisors may be involved either in gathering evidence or in presenting it at the interview.

The Advisory Conciliation and Arbitration Service (ACAS) has produced the following guidelines governing dismissal.

DISCIPLINARY PROCEDURE
A disciplinary procedure should:

1 be in writing
2 specify to whom it applies
3 provide for matters to be dealt with quickly
4 indicate disciplinary actions which may be taken
5 specify the levels of management which have authority to take various forms of disciplinary action, ensuring that immediate superiors do not normally have the power to dismiss without reference to senior management
6 provide for individuals to be informed of the complaints against them and to be given the opportunity to state their case before decisions are reached
7 give individuals the right to be accompanied by a trade union representative or fellow employee of their choice
8 ensure that, except for gross misconduct, no employees are dismissed for a first breach of discipline
9 ensure that disciplinary action is not taken until the case has been carefully investigated
10 ensure that individuals are given an explanation for any penalty imposed
11 provide right of appeal and specify the procedure to be followed.

Grievance procedure

Employees should have a clear route for grievance procedures, and this route should be stated within the organisational policy. The nature of the grievance is incidental: employees should be encouraged – and given every opportunity – to state their particular grievance to the management.

The grievance procedure should clearly indicate:

- that it exists to resolve disputes quickly
- who should be contacted
- what form of evidence is required
- that matters are dealt with confidentially
- that representation is available, and what form this takes.

With the permission of your manager, carry out the following assignment.

Organise a staff meeting at a mutually convenient time. The aim of the meeting is to review the current effectiveness of staff communication and to suggest possible improvements.

At least one week before the meeting, provide those attending with an agenda which states the time the meeting begins and ends, and lists items for inclusion. In addition to your own agenda, invite staff members to add other topics. An agenda might include the following topics:
- handling information
- salon communication
- minimising conflict in the workplace.

At the meeting you – or a designated secretary – will need to make notes so that you can write minutes. If you are chairing the meeting, ensure that all those present are encouraged to contribute. 'Steer' the proceedings so that comments are relevant to the topic under discussion, and be sure not to overrun.

Before moving on to the next topic, remember to summarise the discussion and seek clarification if necessary, so that the proceedings can be accurately minuted.

Remember to retain all materials that you create, for use in your portfolio.

After completing the assignment, answer these questions in your portfolio.

1 What are your organisation's (a) policy, and (b) expectations, in relation to productive working relationships?
2 What is *your* job specification? What does your manager expect of you? What are the limits of your responsibility and authority?
3 What is the job specification of your team?
4 What legislation affects employment?
5 What methods of communication are effective in fostering a good working climate?
6 What are the likely causes of conflict in your workplace?
7 What are your organisation's expectations in relation to standards of work and behaviour?
8 What documents are required, legally or as a matter of company policy, (a) for people in work, and (b) for disciplinary and grievance procedures?

CHAPTER 10

Finance and resources

INTRODUCTION

In this chapter, we consider the factors that contribute to the effectiveness of the business. This is divided into two main areas:

- resources
- productivity.

HUMAN RESOURCES

Hairdressing is a *labour intensive* service industry. It relies solely on the profits generated from the sales of services and treatments to clients. The people that work within a hairdressing salon are therefore an essential part of the business.

In order for a business to succeed, it has to use its human resource to best effect. Staff plans should be flexible to ensure that client demand and the needs of the salon are met. For example:

- both full-time and part-time staff could be used
- more staff will generally be required towards the end of the week
- when salons open six or seven days a week, there needs to be a rota for days off
- there must always be a balance of junior and senior staff
- staff plans should account for holidays, sickness and maternity leave.

TIME RESOURCES

Time is a resource which, although not tangible, is of importance to the financial effectiveness of the business. It affects issues such as pricing structure and staff training.

As the financial income of the salon is largely based on client service, the price structure should reflect the length of time a service takes. For example, a cut and blow dry may have a time allowance of one hour, while a highlighting service may have an allowance of two hours and will be correspondingly more expensive.

Staff training, although beneficial in the long-term, may have hidden costs in terms of time used. A member of staff who is acting as a trainer is not creating any direct income. Development and achievement of training are measured against time limits.

PHYSICAL RESOURCES

The physical resources of a salon include:

- stock
- fixtures and fittings
- utilities (electricity, water and telephones)
- tools and equipment
- space.

Salons cannot function without them, and it is your job to ensure that they are used in the correct manner.

Stock control

The salon supervisor is responsible for maintaining stock control. This involves devising stock systems and allocating staff to stock-monitoring procedures.

The systems that you devise will provide management with information for stock controls. These will deal with:

- reordering stock
- movements of stock
- usage of stock
- shortages of stock
- the safety and security of stock.

Consumables may be used in the salon or sold to clients for home use. Either way, the salon must have enough stock or it won't be able to function.

Products are purchased by the salon in varying quantities, for short-term or long-term availability. To ensure that the products remain usable or saleable, the supervisor must monitor them. She must be aware of:

- shelf-lives
- handling
- losses
- damage.

Stock in storage is a valuable asset to the company. The supervisor is responsible for its management between delivery and use or sale.

Stocktaking

Items for use, such as tools, small pieces of equipment and potentially hazardous chemicals, should be kept in a locked store, the size of which will depend on the size of the salon and its needs. Individual items are accounted for by stocktaking.

Stocktaking at regular intervals provides management with up-to-date information of stock movement. Without regular stocktaking, individual items and product lines could run out, creating a situation in which services and treatments normally offered were not available. This would mean lost profit to the

> **TIP**
>
> When new stock is placed on shelves for sale or use, ensure that old products are brought forward so that they may be used or sold first.

salon, both at the time and later through a damaged reputation.

Every business requires accurate, reliable accounting systems which will:

- categorise products
- monitor usage
- identify shortages
- report damages or defects
- update records.

These guidelines provide the basis for a simple yet effective stock management system.

Product coding

Many salons now use the technology of personal computers to produce management information. Stock control is one of the facilities available in *software systems* for salon management.

Salons turning over large quantities of stock find it helpful to devise coding systems for the products they use and sell. The product's manufacturer, its category, name and size, can all be stored as a single alphanumerical code, the *product code*. These codes can streamline the processes of stock control, monitoring, pricing and tax calculation.

Products received into storage are individually itemised and allocated the relevant product code. The information is then fed into the computer, as is the information that a product has been used or sold. The computer continually recalculates the stock levels, providing management with automated stock control information and printouts for use in manual stocktaking checks.

This coded system is one form of *point-of-sale* (POS) *management*. Another form uses *bar-coding*. The principle here is exactly the same, but the product information is converted into a series of stripes printed on labels or directly on to the product. The bar codes can be read directly by the computer via a scanning bar-code reader, which recognises the product and makes the necessary stock control adjustments.

A bar code

Ordering stock and taking delivery

Products are purchased either directly from the manufacturer or via a wholesaler, on a credit or cash-based agreement. *Credit account* terms are arranged with the supplier, usually on a monthly payment system.

Placing an order

A salon's order may be placed with a company representative, who completes a *purchase order* on the salon's behalf. The purchase order is a paper system documenting all the manufacturer's product listings and categories: this is returned to the company so that the order can be processed and despatched.

Taking delivery

When the stock order arrives at the salon, it will be accompanied by a *delivery note* which will list the items so far despatched and any that are 'to follow', such as items that are temporarily out of stock. The delivery note must be checked against the contents of the consignment, and discrepancies or damage in transit identified before countersigning the order and confirming the delivery. Any discrepancies between the documents should be referred to the management for later adjustment.

The incoming stock should be moved immediately from reception to a secure location away from the working area of the salon. At a convenient time the salon stock systems can be updated and stock put into storage.

After a period of time the supplier will send an *invoice*, a request for payment. Details of the invoice must be checked against the delivery note and the stock actually received.

Choice of stock

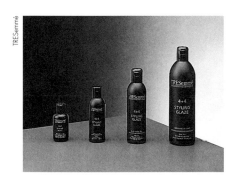

Wholesalers carry stock from a wide range of manufacturers, providing the salon owner with a choice of products and differing prices to suit various budgets. When orders are placed through a manufacturer's representative, however, the salon is restricted to buying the products available from that manufacturer.

You may be able to visit a nearby wholesale 'cash and carry' warehouse. Such warehouses provide an alternative service to the salon, holding stocks ranging from consumable product lines to sundry items such as towels, gowns and hair ornaments, and even coffee and washing powders. Wholesalers like this provide the salon with a 'one-stop' shopping facility.

Stock handling

Most products used by salons are packaged, and many are chemicals. Movements of stock into or within the salon may involve lifting, stacking, dispensing, displaying or pricing, all of which are subject to stringent legislation.

The Health and Safety at Work Act 1974 relates to all workplace health and safety, although the Act has specific requirements for the employer. *Employees* have a duty under the law not to endanger their own health or safety, or that of other people who may be affected by their actions. The responsibilities of the *employer* are summarised below:

- Ensure that the building and the people within it are as safe as possible.
- Train staff in safe working practices and the use of equipment.
- Maintain an accident book and provide first-aid facilities.
- Maintain all equipment and tools.
- Provide safe systems for the handling, transit and storage of all materials.

HEALTH AND SAFETY
If you are unsure about the contents of your salon's products, contact your supplier for relevant COSHH information.

- Implement immediate action when any hazard is reported.
- If the salon employs more than five staff, provide a written health and safety policy describing arrangements for employees.

A specific guide to health and safety in the salon relating to the control of substances hazardous to health (the COSHH regulations) has been written by the Cosmetic, Toiletry and Perfumery Association (CTPA) with the cooperation of the Hairdressing Manufacturers' and Wholesalers' Association (HMWA). This guide assesses substances potentially hazardous to health and provides information to employers about exercising adequate controls.

Apart from basic rules for hairdressers relating to hair products and salon safety, substances are categorised as 'potential' or 'unlikely' hazards. Each type of product identified is specified by:

- name – including ingredients and a general description
- health hazard – from inhalation, ingestion, absorption, contact or injection
- precautions – during work activity, storage, and disposal or spillage
- first aid – in relation to eyes, skin or ingestion
- fire risk – if applicable.

Copies of this guide are available from the HMWA. (For further information, see Chapter 14.)

Security

Stock in storage, as has already been noted, is a valuable asset to the company. Thieves are often opportunist, not always planning their activities: they will seize opportunities as they arise – money left around, products on display, unlocked doors and open windows.

As a supervisor, you should take all necessary precautions to maintain a secure working environment.

Don't:

- leave keys in locks or lying around
- leave products or valuables unattended
- allow unauthorised entry, even by friends or family, to 'staff only' areas.

Do:

- report to management any items that appear to be missing
- ensure that materials and equipment are returned to safe areas
- make available company policy with regard to theft, loss, or damages.

Avoiding waste and damage

Regular checks on goods through careful stock control will assist in minimising shortages, but shortages can still occur if items are neglectfully wasted, such as preparing a colour using a whole tube of tint where half would have been enough. Applications should be carefully measured – manufacturers' recommendations can be found on all products.

Other physical resources can be misused too:

- *Utilities* Staff should be given clear guidelines about the efficient use of utilities, as wastage will increase costs for the salon. For example, taps should not be left on between shampoos; hood dryers should not be left running after the client has finished; and personal calls should not be made from the salon telephones.
- *Tools and equipment* Regular checks on tools and equipment will help minimise problems. These may still occur, however, if items are misused. Using tools for purposes other than those intended could be negligent, if not dangerous. Think of the risks involved in changing a plug using a pair of scissors instead of a screwdriver! Staff must know how to use and maintain tools and equipment in the proper manner, and should be given relevant health and safety training.
- *Space* Effective use of space should also be monitored. Turnover can be measured against the square metre to gauge the productivity of a given area, for example retail sales.

FINANCIAL RESOURCES

In order to make informed decisions about the direction of the business, the owner must have a clear picture of the financial situation. Efficient systems must be put in place to deal with daily financial transactions, and records must be kept so that basic information is available to the salon owner and, as legally required, to Customs and Excise and the Inland Revenue at the end of the financial year.

Financial systems

Company policy will determine the systems and procedures relating to the cashpoint and the format for recording information. These will reflect the line of responsibility. If the salon is a franchise or a concession within a host company, the overall organisation may dictate specific information and presentation requirements, and the salon's manager may be committed to certain obligations built into the business agreement. If the salon stands alone, however, company policy should be established by the owner or manager. It should concern itself with:

- the personnel responsible for cash handling
- the operation of the till (manual, automatic or computerised),

including unders, overs, voids and refunds, and the changing of the till roll
- till reconciliation
- banking
- the recording of information on the daily sheet, in the day book, and in the petty cash book.

The policy should take account of special circumstances which may occur very seldom, if ever:

- *Systems breakdown* What are the procedures in the event of a systems breakdown or power failure? Suppose, for example, you were using an automatic till and it stuck: what would you do? How would you continue to offer service to the client whose transaction you were dealing with?
- *Security* What are the security procedures in the event of fire evacuation? What happens to the takings? Do you lock the till? Who has the key?

Company policy should also determine who is responsible for each function:

- *Line management* What is the line management of a cash transaction? Who is authorised to take money, to process bills, to go to the bank, and to cash up?

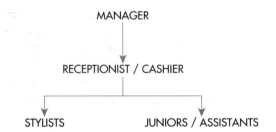

Line management for cash transactions

- *Training* Who is responsible for the delivery and format of training in relation to taking cash and to processing sales? Remember that the training programme needs to be updated to allow for the introduction of new facilities and systems. When a new facility such as an automatic till is introduced into the salon, the company from which it is leased or purchased will usually provide a session of staff training without further charge.

The cashpoint

The systems required at the cashpoint need to be created to match the technical resources. The procedures will therefore differ for manual tills, automatic tills and computerised cash desks.

Manual tills

When operating a manual system, a lockable cashbox or drawer is used to store the cash safely. As the name suggests, a manual system relies upon each transaction being recorded by hand. A daily sheet should itemise each client, with the bill total alongside in the relevant column.

Client	Stylist 1	Stylist 2	Sales
Reynolds	£10.00		
Walker	£12.50		
Davies		£10.00	£5.00

This kind of system can be time-consuming and is the most likely to incur human error.

Automatic tills

Automatic tills are programmed for a number of functions. Each person may be given a code which identifies her takings; this code can be used to calculate commission payments.

On an automatic till, the till roll will display X and Z readings. These readings are used to check the amounts registered against the actual amount in the till. X readings may be used to provide subtotals throughout the day: this is particularly useful in larger companies where it may be helpful to check takings when the cashier or receptionist leaves the till for breaks and for lunch. The Z reading is a figure taken at the close of business for a given day.

Computerised cash desks

Computerised cash desks provide the same facilities as an automatic till but offer many other functions as well. The most important of these functions are the storing and recording of data, and the preparation of management reports.

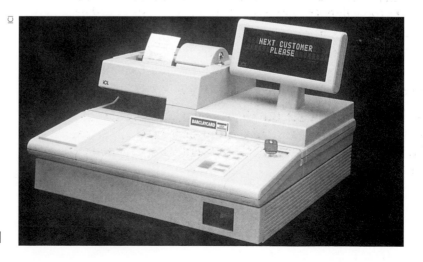

A computerised till

Cashpoint functions

Whichever system is in operation, fundamental procedures are needed to maintain accuracy and efficiency. At all times the person acting as cashier must ensure the client's goodwill.

Float

At the beginning of each working day, the cashpoint must be primed with a float – an amount of money which is surplus to the income from daily transactions. The float amount should be determined from experience, according to the average daily cashflow. It should be made up of the small denominations likely to be required for change.

Method of payment

Payments for sales and services may be made in a number of ways: the salon's house policy will determine what is acceptable.

- *Cash* In Great Britain cash payments will be in pounds sterling, and your salon will probably decline payment in any other currency. Be prepared for unfamiliar coins or notes from other parts of Britain.
- *Cheques* Your salon will probably not accept a cheque unless backed by a *cheque guarantee card*; this will have a limit such as £50 or £100. Company policy may require additional information such as the address of the client and a telephone number. For regular clients you may choose to waive this requirement as a measure of goodwill.
- *Switch/Connect cards* These cards act as automatic cheques: the transaction process is the same as for a cheque or credit card, but once processed the account is debited immediately from the client's bank account.
- *Accounts* Your salon may provide an account facility for regular clients, and a formal arrangement whereby all bills for an individual or a family are paid at agreed intervals. It is advisable to ask the client to sign the bill at the time of service. It should be clear to the stylist when the commission will be paid – either at the time of service or at the time of the account payment.
- *Traveller's cheques* Are these acceptable to your company? If so, in which currencies? Usually traveller's cheques are taken only if they are in sterling. They should be checked against the bearer's passport, for proof of identity.
- *Gift vouchers* Vouchers may be sold by the salon for payment against hairdressing and beauty services or retail sales. When the salon is operating as a concession, gift vouchers may be available for purchase from the host company. You in turn will require reimbursement from the source of the voucher. Company policy should outline procedures for issuing and receiving gift vouchers.

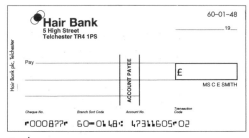

A cheque

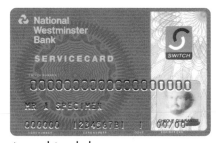

A combined cheque guarantee and switch card

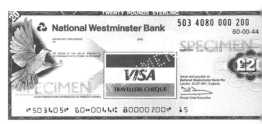

A traveller's cheque, in sterling

A gift voucher

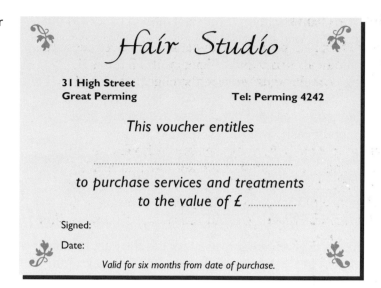

Hair Studio

**31 High Street
Great Perming**
                                    Tel: Perming 4242

This voucher entitles

....

*to purchase services and treatments
to the value of £* ....

Signed:

Date:

Valid for six months from date of purchase.

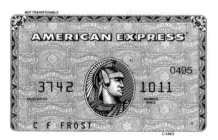

A charge card

- *Credit cards* These cards (such as Access and Visa) may be tendered for payment: upon authorisation from the house company, the amount specified is charged to the cardholder. The salon is charged a percentage on all transactions processed.
- *Charge cards* These cards (such as American Express and Diner's Club) may be tendered for payment in the same way as credit cards. Again, the salon is charged a percentage on all transactions processed.

Card payments

Registered companies may apply to a credit card company to become a *credit card authority*. Upon acceptance of the application, the credit company will issue a transaction machine and the stationery required to make purchase transactions and follow set banking procedures.

Credit cards are accepted as a method of payment at the discretion of the salon. When a card has been accepted as the method of payment, a charge will be imposed by the credit company for the use of this facility.

A list of cards that are accepted by the salon for payment should be clearly displayed. Clients usually presume that payment by card will be acceptable: failure to inform them to the contrary can cause an embarrassing situation to arise. Card payments are given a 'ceiling' limit by the card company: payment will be honoured up to a specific amount; for large amounts prior authorisation by telephone is required. Thorough training needs to be given if staff are to understand these procedures.

Financial records

In order to maintain and analyse the finances of the business, daily records must be completed which will provide weekly, monthly and yearly information. This information can form the basis of development and expansion.

The main purpose of these records is to display two things:

1 cash receipts, and the proportional amount of value-added tax (VAT)
2 the varying expenses paid out – these are usually paid through a petty cash system.

Company policy will determine the layout and systems of records of all daily financial transactions.

Value-added tax (VAT)

VAT is money taken by the business as part of the cost of services and sales, and paid to Customs and Excise: VAT is a percentage added to the total, the percentage being set by the government and changed from time to time. VAT registration is required only for companies whose annual turnover exceeds some current threshold imposed by government.

Day sheets

Cash receipts are recorded in the first instance on a day sheet. This breaks down the total amount of *gross* takings into components, services and sales. The VAT is then calculated from the gross amount and deducted to give the *net* amount. (A 'gross' amount is an amount including VAT.) The purpose of the VAT calculation is to know what proportion of the total takings is usable income.

Example 1: adding VAT

Stylist Graham charges £10 (the net amount) for a cut and blow dry. Assuming VAT is charged at 17.5%:

Net amount	£10.00
Add VAT: 17.5%	+£ 1.75
Gross amount	£11.75

The actual price for a cut and blow dry with Graham is therefore £11.75.

Example 2: deducting VAT

When the amount taken is the *gross* figure, we need to *deduct* the VAT to find the *net* figure. This calculation is more complicated.

In this case we know that the gross amount includes VAT at the current rate. If VAT is charged at 17.5%, the gross amount is 117.5% of the net amount:

Gross amount	£11.75
Deduct VAT: divide by 117.5 and multiply by 17.5*	−£ 1.75
Net amount	£10.00

A day sheet

| STYLIST | SALES | BILL NO. | AMOUNT | TOTAL | | |
				Gross	VAT	Net
	TOTAL					
	EXPENSES					
	TOTAL LESS EXPENSES					
	AMOUNT BANKED					
	PAYING-IN NO.					
	UNDER					
	OVER					

Day .... Date ....

SIGNED ....

(*This is the same as dividing by 47 and multiplying by 7, which you may find simpler.)

Warning Note carefully that this is *not* the same as simply deducting 17.5% of the gross figure:

Gross amount	£11.75	
Deduct 17.5%	£ 2.06	(wrong method)
	£ 9.69	(this result is incorrect)

The day book

The analysis of each day sheet is transferred into a day book. The day book may include other information as well as records of financial transactions.

The basic layout of the book should display the gross amounts taken by each sales and service department, the VAT, and the net takings. This can be totalled weekly, monthly, quarterly, and six-monthly to provide details for precise analysis.

The petty cash book

The petty cash book records each item of expenditure: these amounts will vary. Monies put into petty cash can be from the till, as and when required – these will need to be itemised on the day sheet – or they can be fixed amounts paid in at regular intervals.

A petty cash book

Date	Docket No.	Item	Total amount spent	Amount entered	Milk/Tea Coffee	Stationery	Laundry	Cleaning	Sundries	VAT
4/8				100.00						
4/8		milk	0.39		0.39					
5/8		stamps	4.80						4.80	
6/8		petrol	10.00						8.52	1.48
7/8		envelopes	2.40			2.40				

PRODUCTIVITY

For a hairdressing business to be successful, the salon owner has to take an overall view of productivity. As we have established the business to be mainly labour intensive, there needs to be a continuous analysis of *personal performance* which can only be measured against a *target* figure.

Firstly, the salon owner has to set an overall salon target. This figure can then be divided between departments of stylists, technical and retail. Each person in each department then has a personal target which they understand and agree with.

The personal target can be worked out as follows:

Target = Service price × Number of clients

For example, if stylist Kerry charges £25 for a cut and blow dry and can take 10 clients a day, her daily takings for this service would be £250 and her weekly takings would be £1,250 (based upon a 5-day week). This may be adjusted to allow for different daily performances – we cannot ensure consistent bookings, although through analysis we can establish high and low points. In addition to the styling takings, we would also expect some retail sales, so the overall personal target would include this.

Target setting should follow the SMART principle. It should be:

- *specific* – clearly defined
- *measurable* – quantifiable in some way
- *agreed* – between both parties
- *realistic* – able to be achieved
- *timed* – for the duration of a fixed time period.

Targets may be confidential between the manager and employee, in which case salon procedures relating to confidentiality must be observed. Personal reviews or appraisals provide an opportunity for management to establish an employee's performance level, to compare it against her target, and to discuss ways of improving productivity (see Chapter 9).

Most hairdressing businesses work on a commission basis, which has a strong financial impact on salaries. The salon owner needs to establish fixed costs and variable costs, and the *wage percentage* needs to be established in order for the expected profit level to be achieved. From the overall wage percentage, a target for each stylist is created, allowing for the salaries of 'non-productive' staff such as receptionists and trainees.

ASSIGNMENTS

With the permission of your manager, carry out the following assignments:

1 Create a stock-recording system. The simplest way to devise such a system for your salon is as follows. Armed with a notebook, review the various consumable stock items (the product categories) that your salon purchases. Use a separate page for each category (perms, colours, shampoos, etc.), remembering that certain categories of stock have a range of different types (e.g. perms have normal, tinted and bleached formulations). Provide space to record brand names. Make adjacent columns, headed 'Recommended stock holding level', 'Stock in hand' and 'Stock on order'.

2 Document daily payment transactions, breaking the payments down into services and sales and itemising cash and non-cash payments. Carry out the VAT calculation. Continue this for one month, to give records suitable for analysis.

3 Create a petty-cash recording system for use on a daily basis. Use it for one month and analyse the evidence produced.

4 List the pros and cons of using each of the following cash facilities:
   • manual
   • automatic till
   • computerised cashpoint.

Using the above assignments as guidance, make notes on your work, ensuring that you document all of the aspects of financial control. Remember to keep examples of the systems or materials that you create, for use in your portfolio.

QUESTIONS

After completing the assignments, answer these questions in your portfolio.

1 What are your company's procedures for stocktaking?

2 What levels of stocks does your organisation hold?

3 What are the possible causes of product deterioration or damage? What action should you take?

4 What information is required for simple book-keeping purposes?

5 How is VAT calculated?

6 What VAT is payable on £10? What VAT has been included if the *gross* amount is £10?

7 What problems could occur during day-to-day till operations?

8 What action does your salon take when anomalies occur during the day-to-day till operations?

9 What is your company's policy for dealing with abnormal situations such as unexplained losses?

CHAPTER 11

Training

INTRODUCTION

This chapter looks at the training and development of salon personnel. It considers the following functions:

- identifying training needs
- planning training
- delivering training
- supporting training
- self-development.

THE PROVISION OF TRAINING

The success or failure of any business is dependent on the individual skills of the personnel. To meet the changing demands caused by commercial pressures, it is vital that training takes place for all employees at whatever level. Employees need:

- to increase their knowledge
- to develop their skills
- to carry out their job more effectively than before.

Sources of training

To achieve the training objectives, groups or individuals may utilise a variety of sources:

- college-based programmes
- private training organisations
- government schemes and initiatives
- manufacturers' courses
- salon-based training.

These sources of training may involve a number of learning methods and techniques, which fall into two categories:

- directed learning
- student-centred learning.

For example, training workshops and classroom methods involve individuals who train, coach and support the learner: this style of delivery is *directed learning*. On the other hand, specially designed projects and assignments, open learning and correspondence courses may involve private study: although such study may be

> **TIP**
>
> Useful sources of information for updating skills include product manufacturers, the trade press, local colleges and the Hairdressing Training Board.

supported by a field tutor, this type of learning is referred to as *student-centred*.

TIP

People respond to different types of training – explore these and find which methods suit which learners.

Types of training

Choosing the type or style of training is probably the most important factor in devising a training programme. Effective training is 'tailormade' to suit the learner. Valuable time, money and effort is wasted if the programmes devised do not meet the needs of the learner.

Imagine that you are a salon trainer, trying to instruct a trainee in how to shampoo correctly. You may have a shampooing system specific to your salon, which lists the various stages within the procedure:

1 Prepare and protect the client with a clean gown and towel.
2 Check that the client is comfortable.
3 Brush through to disentangle the client's hair.
4 Select and prepare the correct shampoo.
5 Check the water temperature and pressure . . .

Clearly it would be pointless to teach such a procedure by means of a printed list if the trainee had reading difficulties. Similarly, to maximise the effectiveness of any training you need to evaluate the training *needs* of the learner. Then, depending on these findings, and subject to your company's budgetary constraints, choose the most suitable type of training.

Workshops

Workshops are the ideal mechanism for the group training of practical hairdressing skills. Utilising the salon environment, a trainer can demonstrate techniques, guide the learners either on 'live' models or on practice blocks, and monitor their progress.

Demonstrations

The 'look and learn' technique of a demonstration can be used effectively to impart technical expertise or procedures, such as the step-by-step process of precision fashion cutting.

The demonstrator should not try to cram in too much information. There must be ample time, and the demonstrator should be prepared to answer any questions. In this approach there is little audience participation.

Presentations and seminars

Presentations and seminars are often used as informative, instructional sessions. They can be enjoyable, but only if the presenter is fully prepared and competent in presentation techniques – if not, the audience may lose interest and miss key points.

If you prefer to use this style for your training, remember these guidelines:

- Keep the session as short as possible.
- Divide your presentation into logical steps, each containing 'digestible' chunks of information.
- Refocus your audience's attention from time to time by summarising key points.

Role-play

Role-plays are simulations of activities carried out by individuals or groups. They are often used in the development of communication skills and customer care, for instance for reception techniques. The trainer observes and facilitates the learners by prompting or by giving constructive feedback. Role-plays can be video-recorded, so that the learners may review their own performance.

Role-play helps learners to adapt their skills to different situations, such as handling difficult clients, dealing with complaints, or taking part in staff disciplinary action.

Flexible learning

In flexible learning, the learner uses a variety of training materials – text-based, computer-based, video- and audio-taped – to teach herself at a distance from the training centre. Support and guidance are offered.

> **TIP**
> There are a variety of materials available for flexible learning – contact your local college for help.

IDENTIFYING TRAINING NEEDS

The most obvious indication of a need for training is an individual's (or a team's) inability to carry out a job. If a hair stylist shows reluctance to undertake certain services, such as setting or working with long hair, this may indicate that she lacks the required skills or confidence, or both.

Poor performances that indicate a need for training fall into the following functional areas:

- operational systems
- communications
- service quality
- selling
- health and safety.

Below are lists of typical tasks that are often 'underperformed' in the salon. You may like to use these as checklists within your own work environment.

Operational systems

1 Till transactions
2 Procedures for daily/weekly financial accounting
3 Client service/treatment records

4 Appointment scheduling
5 Stock management

Communications

1 Telephone techniques
2 Customer enquiries
3 Client consultations
4 Handling complaints
5 External business contacts
6 Staff communications

Service quality

1 Standards of technical ability
2 Standards of professionalism
3 Client care

Selling

1 Retailing products
2 Services and treatments
3 Aftercare sales (between visits)
4 Yourself

Health and safety

1 Salon hygiene
2 Personal hygiene
3 Client health and safety
4 Staff health and safety
5 Maintenance of tools and equipment

PLANNING TRAINING

Before you can put together a training plan, you need to have a defined aim, which will be met by clear objectives. Use the following questions to identify the key training factors. Try to answer each of the questions in clear concise statements: this will help you to piece together an outline for a training plan.

- *What* is the purpose of the training?
- *Who* are the trainees?
- *How* will the desired outcome be achieved?
- *When* will training take place?
- *Where* will training take place?

These simple questions will help you focus on the *objectives* (the desired outcomes). After devising the framework of the training plan, you can then consider the other factors (the *inputs*).

The aim

- The training purpose

The objectives

Are the objectives:

- knowledge-based
- practical skills
- a combination of both?

The resources

What resources will be necessary:

- time
- money
- equipment
- people
- venue?

The delivery technique

What are the most efficient methods for delivering the training:

- workshops
- demonstrations
- presentations
- role-play
- flexible learning?

The assessment

How will you know when the objective has been achieved:

- observing performance
- oral questioning
- written testing?

The monitoring

How will you check for continuing knowledge or skill retention:

- coaching
- reviews
- meetings?

When you have evaluated and documented answers to all of these key factors, your simple outline plan will have expanded into a detailed training programme.

DELIVERING TRAINING

If you are the designated trainer, responsible for training others in your organisation, you will have to consider the necessary preparations of:

- the training session
- the trainee or trainees
- yourself.

The training session

Regardless of whether you are making a presentation to an audience of 50 people or demonstrating a new colouring technique to an individual, you need to be adequately prepared to impart the knowledge or skill.

The simplest way of preparing the session is to produce a list of points to include and things to think about, under the following headings:

The aim

To provide a quality, preparatory service to the customer

The objective

To train others to competence in shampooing clients in preparation for future services or treatments

The resources

(a) Model for shampooing
(b) Suitable products
(c) Available work area
(d) Clean gowns, towels, etc.

The training techniques

(a) Demonstrate skills/procedures
(b) Discuss client communications
(c) Product awareness
(d) Promote feedback
(e) Observe trainee(s) practising

The assessment

(a) Observe performance
(b) Verify actions by questioning
(c) Make assessment decision
(d) Feedback to trainee(s)

Trainees

With the session planned, you must then prepare the trainees. Ensure that the trainees are:

- available at the allotted time and place
- aware of what is required of them
- ready with any other required materials
- prepared to ask questions
- guided and supported throughout the session.

Yourself

When you have carried out the procedures outlined above, you will be almost ready to implement the training. The final step is preparing yourself. Provided that you have the necessary skills and knowledge, the training activity should be straightforward.

One good way of focusing on the expected activities during the programme is to produce a *training schedule*. This is a paper plan outlining the requirements:

- objectives
- resources and equipment
- duration
- tutor/trainer activity
- trainees' activities
- knowledge and skill inputs
- method for testing objectives.

A training schedule

Objective	Shampooing in preparation for further services	
Equipment	Gown, towels, brushes, combs, products	
Resources	Writing materials, text materials	
Duration	30 minutes	

	Trainer activity	Trainee activity	Training content
1	Prepare and protect client	Observe procedure	Health and safety (client)
2	Check water temperature and pressure	Feel temperature and correct pressure	Health and safety (client)
3	Select suitable products (explain benefits)	Observe and make notes	Product knowledge
4	Demonstrate procedure	Observe procedure	Method/technique
5	Prompt trainees for questions	Ask questions	Underpinning knowledge

Method for testing the objective

6	Observe and guide trainee	Practise shampoo procedure	Method/technique
7	Question trainee	Respond to questions (oral/written)	Underpinning knowledge

SUPPORTING LEARNERS

If trainers simply present knowledge and skills without supporting or guiding the learner, very few trainees will reach competence. The 'sink or swim' approach to training often used in the past imposed a 'survival of the fittest' attitude. Trainees who have not been offered support during their training often feel isolated and insecure in their work: they tend to lack confidence, motivation and ability.

The trainer should always give positive support and constructive feedback to the trainee, during or after training sessions – *even* if performance has been poor. This helps the trainee to 'build' on skills she already has. By guiding and supporting the trainee in this way, the trainer will be able to monitor progress and identify individual strengths and weaknesses. This will enable the trainer to:

- review the trainee's progress
- produce personal training plans
- devise suitable action plans
- evaluate the effectiveness of the training.

Personal action or training plans

Personal training plans (PTPs) and personal action plans (PAPs), completed by the trainee with assistance from the trainer, are ideal tools for:

- providing agreed, personalised training targets
- providing training time scales
- specifying individual training requirements
- stating dates for formal review.

An example of a plan is provided on the following page. The columns are used as follows:

1 Training topic – e.g. 11.1 Demonstration of skills and methods to learners.
2 Training (Trg.) – a tick in this column shows that training for this activity is required.
3 Experience (Exp.) – a tick in this column shows that further experience or practice is required.
4 Action to be taken.
5 The agreed date for completion of the activity.
6 The agreed date for review of progress.

Personal Action Plan

| Candidate name | | Jane Smith | | | Date 12/8/97 |

Unit and element	Trg.	Exp.	Action(s) required	Target date	Review date
Unit II Element II.I	✓		TRAINING ACTIVITY I will: 1 Devise an assessment plan for an individual involving natural performance, covering 4 elements of competence 2 Describe how the plan meets the performance criteria 3 Provide oral evidence that I have covered the range and related knowledge	22/11/97	29/11/97

SELF-DEVELOPMENT

Do you 'practise what you preach'? Always, usually, sometimes, seldom, or never?

If you had to think about your answer for more than a few seconds, you did not answer 'always'! So could it also be said that you don't lead by example? Don't worry – this isn't a personal failing, just human nature.

Motivation is the key. It is how we motivate others and ourselves that makes targets attainable. Imagine that you needed to do something that you didn't feel like doing. What would make you do it: an incentive, to encourage you; or a threat, so that you responded out of dislike or fear? Most people would prefer the incentive approach, which channels the effort in a controlled, systematic forward movement.

In seeking to develop yourself in your work, you cannot just rely on management to define the targets and monitor the performance. You must motivate yourself to set useful, achievable objectives. This form of positive, active participation will help lead to:

- better working relationships
- increased job satisfaction
- greater self-esteem
- improved efficiency.

Self-appraisal

Identify your own strengths and weaknesses. One way of doing this is to use the existing NVQ standards, incorporating performance criteria, range and essential knowledge as a checklist, to see where competence has been or can be achieved (see Chapter 9, pages 159–60).

Self-discipline

Maintaining the diligence, determination and self-motivation to see a task through to a satisfactory conclusion requires a lot of self-discipline. Without this quality you will not achieve your goals.

Self-organisation

Use your organisational skills to plan an effective route to your objectives. Develop your time management so that you focus on tasks that *have* to be performed – letters, reports, work schedules, and so on. Devise lists of things to do, putting them in order of priority. Remove items when you have completed the tasks. With your manager, evaluate the effectiveness of your performance.

ASSIGNMENT

With the permission of your manager, carry out the following assignment.

1 Identify the training needs for individual staff members in your salon. Select appropriate staff to undergo training activities. After discussions with each trainee involved, identify relevant activities (elements) from Hairdressing Level 2.

   Devise personal training programmes to meet each trainee's needs, including suitable time scales.

2 Draft session plans to meet the objectives and deliver the training.

3 After the training has been delivered, evaluate its success. This should be carried out with the trainees, documenting their comments so that you can review the effectiveness of the training activities later.

Keep the training programmes, session plans and evaluations, for use in your portfolio.

QUESTIONS

After completing the assignment, answer these questions in your portfolio.

1 How do you (a) analyse, (b) evaluate, and (c) present information?

2 What is your own role within your company in respect to training? What authority and autonomy do you have?

3 List the most effective methods for providing communication (a) between staff, and (b) between you and your manager.

4 Describe techniques that can be used for self-appraisal.

CHAPTER 12

Assessment

INTRODUCTION

This chapter looks at the assessment and reporting of training outcomes. It considers the following functions:

- identifying assessment opportunities
- assessing practical skill
- assessing underpinning knowledge
- recording competence and providing feedback.

STANDARDS OF COMPETENCE

The Hairdressing Training Board's current nationally recognised standards for hairdressing are the product of close liaison between the industry representatives from a variety of hairdressing employer associations, artistic creative groups, and training organisations. With assistance from external training consultants, the hairdressing industry has been able to devise appropriate standards to meet the needs of the profession, while maintaining the requirements of the Qualifications and National Curriculum Authority (QCA).

Before NVQs were available, students wishing to gain qualifications in hairdressing practised and studied in line with a syllabus. After they had completed the course, they took practical and theoretical examinations. Depending on how they performed on the day, they either passed or failed.

Now students who attend approved training programmes participate in *continual assessment*: they practise the required skills; they learn the relevant background knowledge; and at the point at which they can perform tasks consistently to the set standard, they are deemed competent.

At some time, we have all heard comments referring to standards: 'Our high street salon has higher standards than those on the estates' or 'This college expects the highest standards from the students.' Without explanation of what these standards are, such statements are meaningless.

To achieve nationally recognised standards within any given task, such as 'cutting hair into a uniform layered shape', the learner must reach and maintain the required skill and knowledge; and the assessor must be able to measure accurately the level of competence, so that the candidate has access to fair assessment.

Components of standards

A standard is a written specification of how a task or function should be performed. It has the following components:

- an element title
- performance criteria
- range statements
- essential knowledge.

'Assessing to standard' is a way of using the information contained within these key components either as a checklist or as a framework from which questions may be devised that will highlight expertise or knowledge in a particular situation or conditions.

Element title

An individual standard is called an *element*. The title of an element states the function or task that has to be performed, for example 'Element 2.2 Restyle hair to create a variety of looks'.

Each specific area of work will consist of more than one activity or task. These tasks, when grouped together, are called *units*. 'Unit 2 Apply cutting techniques to create a variety of looks', for instance, is made up of two elements of competence, as illustrated below.

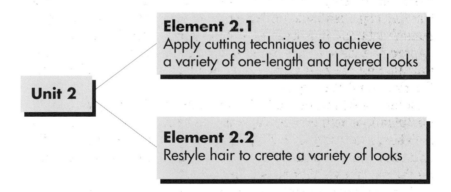

Unit 2

Element 2.1
Apply cutting techniques to achieve a variety of one-length and layered looks

Element 2.2
Restyle hair to create a variety of looks

Level 3 in hairdressing comprises thirteen units of competence. Six of these units are compulsory. A further five units are optional, but at least three must be undertaken to achieve Level 3 in hairdressing. In addition, there are two units for assessment which are taken at the candidate's discretion. Candidates may accumulate units:

- for specific areas of work-related tasks
- for part certification
- for full Level 3 certification
- in any order
- at their own pace of learning
- within the workplace or at a training centre.

Occupational Standard
Unit 2 Apply cutting techniques to create a variety of looks

Element 2.1
Apply cutting techniques to achieve a variety of one length and layered looks

---

Performance criteria

a) preparation of client is in accordance with salon requirements and client wishes regarding the look to be achieved are confirmed

b) own decisions regarding the combination and application of cutting techniques are based on maximising the potential of the client's hair

c) tools and equipment selected are suitable for achieving the required look

d) attention is paid to detail throughout the cutting process, taking into account critical influencing factors

e) the application of cutting techniques is creative and results in achievement of the required look

f) hair is finished creatively to complement the cut

g) the finished look is to the satisfaction of the client and enhances own professional image and that of the salon

---

Range statements

i) One length and layered looks are achieved on hair that is:
  - curly
  - wavy
  - straight

ii) Cutting techniques:
  - graduating
  - club-cutting
  - scissor and clipper over comb
  - thinning – with scissors or razor
  - freehand
  - tapering
  - texturising

iii) Finishing techniques:
  - drying
  - product application

iv) Critical influencing factors:
  - client wishes
  - hair texture
  - head and face shape
  - hair growth pattern
  - hair movement

Essential knowledge and understanding requirements

- Ways in which cutting and finishing techniques can be combined and applied to best effect
- Importance of paying attention to detail and how critical factors can influence the cutting of hair
- Significance of satisfying the client
- Professional image of the salon and the benefits to be gained by enhancing it
- Health and safety considerations which must be taken into account when cutting hair

Level 3 Element

Performance criteria

A standard specifies not only *what* has to be done, but also *how* it is to be done: the performance criteria. Performance criteria are lists of concise statements of procedural functions. These must be followed, in order. For example, 'The candidate must: (a) make small neat sections; (b) check shape and balance; (c) hold the hair at the appropriate angle', and so on. These performance criteria are used as a checklist when the candidate is being observed during assessment.

Range

If a trainee were asked to perform a uniform, layered haircut on a model with straight hair, the finished cut would not appear the same as the same cut carried out on a model with curly hair: although the same techniques and skills are required in both situations, the outcome would be very different. This range of contexts – type, length, texture and the like – yields a wide variety of conditions which may affect the task.

Essential knowledge

In the case of the candidate performing a uniform haircut on straight hair, it is clear that she should have sufficient background knowledge about suitability of hairstyles, types of hair and their styling properties, growth patterns, final effects and so forth, if she is to work competently. This background knowledge underpins the practical task and is essential to the operation.

ASSESSING TRAINEES

It is the continual monitoring of training and work experience that leads to assessment. Your informed decisions relating to trainees' capabilities can only be recorded as:

- competent
- not yet competent
- insufficient evidence to judge competence.

Awards of merit – 'pass with credit', 'pass with merit', 'distinction' and the like – do not exist within NVQs.

Why do we assess?

1 To check whether a trainee can perform her job competently.
2 To check where a trainee can improve.
3 To record progress towards achievement.
4 To record achievement.

How do we assess?

1 Performance is assessed by observation.
2 Knowledge is assessed by oral and written means.

Recognising an assessment opportunity

The decision that it is time to assess can come from the trainer, from the trainee, or – by mutual agreement – from both. Knowing *when* to assess is the most important stage within the monitoring process.

Monitoring performance towards competence will occur during:

- normal work routines
- formal training activities
- role-plays and simulations.

Performance can be judged by the most appropriate assessment methods of those listed below:

- live observation
- observation of video-recordings
- discussion with the trainee
- discussion with other informed personnel
- examination or review of records, plans, assignments, projects, case studies, and the like.

TIP

Encourage trainees to monitor their own performance. Make copies of the standards available to them so that they can use the performance criteria as a checklist.

Collecting evidence

To gain proof of a trainee's competence, you must use a combination of the three evidence collection systems available: observation, oral and written. Assessors should give the trainee constructive feedback and record the outcomes, directly after the assessment process and on the appropriate documentation.

Naturalistic assessment

Watching natural performance is probably the most reliable basis for skill assessment. When trainees are carrying out their normal day-to-day routines, the trainer/assessor can unobtrusively monitor their progression. Ongoing informal assessment will show quite clearly whether trainees have retained previously learned skills.

Competence in a given activity on a single occasion is seldom sufficient evidence to infer 'occupational' competence – most practical activities must be observed during several performances before they can be documented in the trainee's record of achievement (the 'summative assessment' record).

Pre-arranged assessment

Formal observation usually takes place during training activities. When candidates are required to be formally assessed, they should be made aware of the assessment conditions beforehand. They need to know:

- what is required of them
- what it is they are to perform
- what additional preparations are necessary.

Trade tests, skill tests and role-play simulations may be situations in which formal observation is necessary.

Remember: for you to know whether the candidate has performed to the *minimum* standard, you must use the performance criteria as a checklist for your assessment.

Oral questioning

Oral assessment should always take place immediately after the practical performance. Oral questions are devised by the assessor and framed around the work being carried out. The purpose of oral questioning is to test the knowledge of the candidate and the actions she would take:

- in a range of different situations
- to allow for unforeseen circumstances.

In structuring oral questions, bear in mind that questions may be either 'open' or 'closed'. *Open questions* are used to invite detailed information. They usually begin with words such as 'How', 'Why', 'When', 'Where' or 'What'. Examples are 'Why should you use end papers when winding a perm?' and 'When should you take a test curl during perming?' *Closed questions* are used when only a simple 'yes' or 'no' response is required. For example, 'Should you carry out a skin test before colouring a client's hair?'

It is up to the assessor to decide when is the best time to ask questions. In general, if the task is complex or intricate it may be better to wait until the activity has been completed. Tasks that involve breaks, such as processing times during chemical operations, provide natural opportunities for questions.

Written assessment

Written questions are generally used some time *after* the practical activity has been carried out. They should be constructed in such a way as to allow you to assess essential knowledge that would not normally be assessed orally. (Background knowledge that affects the health, safety or security of clients and staff should be tested *before* the activity is performed.)

The drawback with written questions is that they may put the candidate under pressure. For this reason, another form of popular written evidence is the *portfolio* (see Appendix 1).

Recorded evidence

The term 'recorded evidence' relates to numerous additional forms of alternative evidence which together provide a permanent record: reports, documents or illustrations. However it is produced, it must be attributed to the candidate. (Examples of recorded evidence may be found in Appendix 1.)

PROVIDING FEEDBACK

After the performance has been assessed, it is essential to provide the candidate with feedback relating to her level of ability and competence. Assessments are judged with strict adherence to the standards (the elements). It is therefore very important to discuss these findings on a one-to-one basis with the candidate.

The feedback given should be constructive, positive and

supportive, regardless of whether the candidate has failed on this occasion. Often candidates fail to meet the standards because of simple errors or omissions. These need to be clearly identified and understood. This will enable the candidate to reach the expected level of competence on a subsequent occasion.

The feedback will vary from assessor to assessor, candidate to candidate, depending on individual needs. It is important for the assessor to adapt the feedback to meet these needs.

During the feedback to the candidate, or shortly afterwards, the candidate's personal record of assessment must be completed. Accurate records are an integral part of the assessment process, and these must be kept and made available for verification purposes.

ASSIGNMENT

With the permission of your manager, carry out the following assignment using the applicable current standards:

1 Assess trainees' performance and underpinning knowledge. (Ideally, this should form a continuation assignment following the key assignment for training.)

Following discussion with the trainees, devise personal assessment plans with suitable time scales. Devise suitable oral and written questions, framed around the essential knowledge requirements from the elements to be assessed.

After assessments have been made, give feedback to the trainees on their individual performances.

2 Record the assessment outcomes within the appropriate trainee records.

Keep copies of the assessment plans, the questions you devised and the trainee records for use in your portfolio.

QUESTIONS

After completing the assignment, answer these questions in your portfolio.

1 What details have you documented in respect of your staff's agreed training plans and objectives?

2 What conditions and which situations provide ideal opportunities for collecting assessment evidence?

3 What are effective methods for communication and negotiation?

4 What constitutes satisfactory performance evidence?

5 To whom would you refer if you had difficulties in interpreting performance criteria?

6 What constitutes satisfactory evidence of knowledge?

7 How and when should oral questions be used?

8 What additional requirements might candidates with special needs have?

9 What constitutes sufficient evidence of competence?

10 How do you record assessment information?

11 How would you provide feedback to a candidate after making your assessment decisions?

CHAPTER 13

Salon promotion

INTRODUCTION

This chapter looks at ways in which a salon can enhance its profile and encourage increased sales of the services offered. Your salon may already organise some form of promotion, for example a colour or perm 'sale'. During a quiet time, when the salon takings are expected to be at their lowest, offering a discounted price for colouring or for a perm may attract new clients to the salon, thereby increasing revenue. However, there are also other forms of promotion that your salon might want to consider, including demonstrations and advertising.

PROMOTING THE BUSINESS

In order to promote your services, you need to recognise how they are perceived by prospective clients. To do this you need to consider each service in terms of its features and its benefits:

- *features* are the functions – what the service does
- *benefits* are the results of the functions – what the service achieves.

For example, suppose you hope to persuade a client to spend £20 on a cut and blow dry. Why should she do so? What are the benefits of the service? The *feature* is a precision cut. The *benefits* are keeping shape and easier home styling. The client must decide whether the payment of £20 is justified by these benefits.

Consider a second example: application of a semi-permanent colour. In this case the *features* are that the colour is not permanent and is applied in a conditioning base. The *benefits* are that it will wash out after 6–8 shampoos, and meanwhile it will create shine.

Knowledge of service and product features enables you to sell your clients the benefits. You thereby create a need, and once the client has accepted the need, you are in a good position to make the sale.

The first step is therefore to gain a thorough knowledge of each service and product available in the salon, and to convert this knowledge into a recognition of the features and benefits in each case. The next step is to inform the potential market by means of promotion.

Successful promotion requires careful planning. Time and thought need to be given to each aspect.

Identify the objectives

What do you want the promotion to achieve? Is it to attract new clients, for example, or to increase colours or perms, or to increase retail sales?

Whatever the objectives, it is most effective always to concentrate the promotion on a *single* aim.

Decide on the type of promotion

There are many possibilities – here are a few:

- offering an introductory discount to new clients
- offering a service with another service, for example a complementary conditioning treatment with colouring
- introducing a retail product, for example offering a free retail conditioner for permed hair with each perm treatment
- implementing an incentive scheme for staff who reach sales targets in product sales and treatments
- demonstrating your services through a 'hair show', either at the salon or at a venue chosen to suit the target group.

Prepare promotional activities

It is best to write an outline or plan of your promotion. From that you will be able to identify each area requiring preparation.

Order stock and promotional materials

You may need to have leaflets printed or place an advertisement to inform potential clients. You may need additional materials: for instance, for a perm promotion you will need to order additional perms. (Most product houses will provide advice and merchandising support.)

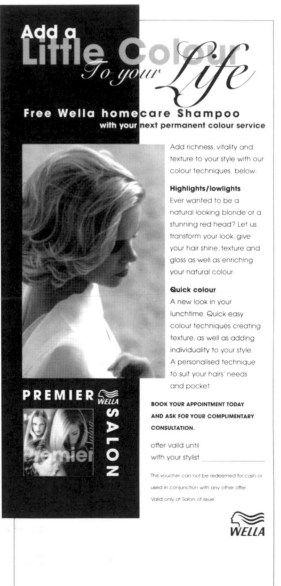

A promotional leaflet

Inform staff

Ensure that all staff are fully aware of the promotion. This may require refresher training, for example in product knowledge. Your presentation to the staff needs to make them enthusiastic: they will then be able to 'sell' the idea to clients.

Inform your target

Select the best medium of communication. You may inform clients verbally. You may try a mailshot, distribute leaflets, display posters or notices, or advertise in local papers or selected magazines. In any written literature, remember to highlight the features and benefits of the service.

Monitor the outcome against the identified objectives

After the promotion, evaluate its success by monitoring your business. If you have been successful, sales will have increased.

You may find that promoting a specific service – perming, for example – will generate an increase in salon revenue overall. This is obviously good in itself, but to obtain the true result of the promotion, the increased business should be set against the initial objective. Thus, if the aim of the promotion were to increase the number of perms during February, you would need to know exactly how many clients had perms in that month, and how many you would have expected *without* the promotion.

Recording promotions

Date: ....

Promotional Outline: ....

Date: .... Leaflets Mailshot (No.) ....
                                          Posters (No.) ....
                                          Advertisement (Type/Place): ....

Leaflets Returned: Week ending: .... No. ....
                        Week ending: .... No. ....
                        Week ending: .... No. ....
                        Week ending: .... No. ....

New Clients Recorded:

Revenue Increases: Cutting: .... %
                        Colour: .... %
                        Perm: .... %
                        Sales: .... %
                        Beauty: .... %

Comments: ....
....
Overall Success Rating: ....

Document the results

To make full use of the promotion result, you need to keep a permanent record of the facts. This record can then be referred to later; gradually you will identify strengths and weaknesses and be able to repeat or amend the promotion, depending upon the results.

DEMONSTRATING SERVICES

Hairdressing demonstrations form a very important part in training and promotion. Displays, both of the skill of the hairdresser's technique and the finished style that she produces, provide opportunities for increasing sales. Informally, of course, every person working in the salon is continually demonstrating their skills from shampooing through to technical services, but there is also a place for the formal demonstration.

To organise a demonstration, you again need to keep to a structure in your planning.

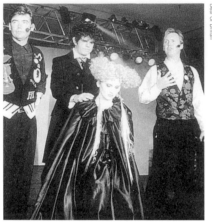

A hair show and demonstration

Identify the objectives

What is the *purpose* of the demonstration? Is it, for example, staff training or salon promotion?

Prepare the resources

What resources do you need? How many people do you expect to attend?

Select the venue

Is the demonstration going to be carried out in the salon, or at a local hall or hotel?

- Will the audience be able to see the demonstration area? Are lighting and sound provided? Can you make use of a raised platform or stage, panoramic mirrors, or revolving hydraulic chairs?
- Are shampooing and dressing facilities available?
- Do you need to arrange transport to the venue for your models and equipment?
- Is the venue easily accessible to your audience by public transport? Are there parking facilities?
- Will you offer refreshments?

Set the budget

You may have a budget available within salon expenditure. If not, you can charge for tickets to pay for your expenses.

To calculate the ticket price, you need to divide your total expenses by the number of people you *expect* to attend (not the number you *hope* will attend!). For example, if your expenses total £500 for an expected audience of 50, the ticket price will be £10. You will need to sell 50 tickets to cover your costs – if you sell more, of course, you will make a small profit.

Your costs need to include:

- the fee for your guest artist, where applicable
- payments to models
- payments to a make-up artist or clothes stylist, where applicable
- the hire of the venue
- the hire of lighting, sound and equipment
- transport costs
- the cost of refreshments for demonstrators, models and the audience
- marketing costs, including advertising and the printing of tickets and programmes
- staff costs, either in salary or the cost to the salon of giving time in lieu.

Plan the demonstration

Consider the model, the content, the method and the explanation.

Depending on the scale of the demonstration, you may need to build in opportunities for the audience to participate and ask questions. This is not possible when demonstrating to a very large number of people, but good communication skills are always essential in creating a rapport with your audience.

Expect the unexpected

To maintain control of the event, your preparation needs to include contingency plans in the event of things going wrong. For example, what would you do:

- if your model did not arrive on time?
- if your guest artist was delayed?
- if there was a power failure?
- if there was a security evacuation?
- if you did not achieve your desired result?

Give thought to each component of the event, and be mentally prepared for any eventuality. You will then feel confident, and your demonstration will be a success.

Make a time schedule

Once you have planned the event, it is advisable to make a

checklist with a time schedule. To do this, start with the event time and work backwards. For example:

6.00 p.m.	The event. Guest artist will demonstrate the latest long hair fashion.
5.30 p.m.	Facility open to the audience.
5.00 p.m.	Final check: platform, demonstration chair, lighting, microphone/sound. Feed models and platform artist.
4.30 p.m.	Check platform tools and equipment. Prepare tray: this should contain everything that the artist will use during her demonstration. Check that all sprays work. [For a cutting demonstration it is a good idea to include a plaster – even the best hairdressers cut their fingers occasionally!]
3.30 p.m.	Model to be made-up.
3.00 p.m.	Arrival of make-up artist.
2.00 p.m.	Arrival of model and guest artist.
12.00 noon	Organiser to arrive at venue. Arrange eating; erect display material. Check preparation area.

Alongside this schedule, make a checklist of each item needed or the event. Remember, planning ahead ensures smooth running.

ADVERTISING

Advertising is always a useful way of promoting your salon's services. It is important to define the purpose of the advertisement so that you can choose the most appropriate form of advertising.

- Do you want to attract new customers?
- Do you want to advertise a new service?
- Do you want to increase the salon's profile?
- Do you want to increase retail sales?
- Do you want to maintain loyalty with regular customers?
- Do you want to draw customers' attention to other services on offer?

There are many different forms of advertising, including:

- magazines
- newspapers
- directories
- leaflets/posters
- local radio
- calendars.

Advertising can be very expensive. Therefore, the form of advertising you choose will also depend on the budget available.

If you decide to advertise your business through printed media, careful consideration must be given to the content of the message you wish to convey (see also section on photography below).

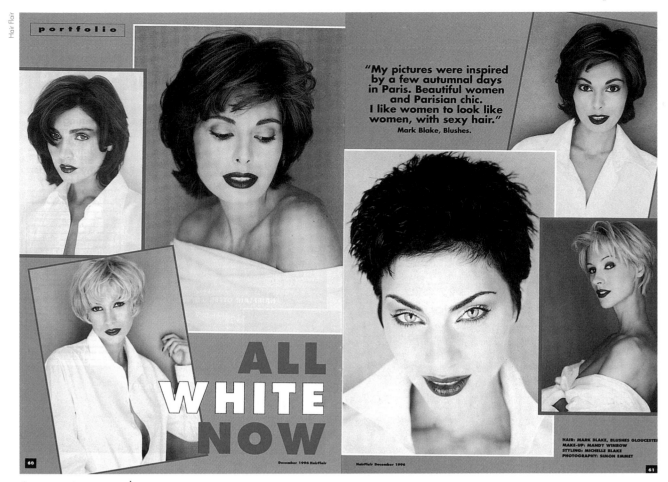

portfolio

"My pictures were inspired by a few autumnal days in Paris. Beautiful women and Parisian chic. I like women to look like women, with sexy hair."
Mark Blake, Blushes.

ALL WHITE NOW

December 1996 HairFlair

HairFlair December 1996

HAIR: MARK BLAKE, BLUSHES GLOUCESTER
MAKE-UP: MANDY WINROW
STYLING: MICHELLE BLAKE
PHOTOGRAPHY: SIMON EMMET

60

61

A magazine spread

PHOTOGRAPHY

Good photography is a very powerful medium. It will instantly convey a message about the type of work you do and the image that you portray as a company. However, professional photo-shoots are a costly option and can be unsuccessful if they are not properly coordinated. Like all other business strategies, professional photography must be well planned.

Identify the objectives

Make sure you understand the purpose of the photo-shoot.

- Is it to attract more customers?
- Is it to exhibit your work?
- Is it for use in the local press or nationally published magazines?

If you are promoting the business through local papers, you will need to bear in mind the quality of print output that the newspaper company can produce. It is hardly worth spending lavishly on professional models, photography and make-up artists if the quality of work and art direction is going to be devalued by the quality of the printed result.

However, if you decide to produce work for magazines, they will expect only high-quality photographic transparencies for their printing processes. Ensuring that your work gets included is down to good PR. Whether you want to handle this yourself or employ the expertise of a public relations agent is up to you, but you will need to produce a *press release* with some news angle if it is to have any chance of being published. In recent years magazines have apportioned more space to health and hair care topics, so the opportunities are improving. In any event, research will have to be done to ensure that any press release produced is received into the right hands.

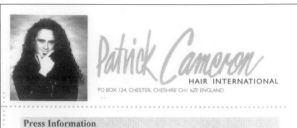

A press release

Define your look (art direction)

- Will your look be classic, fashionable, avant-garde or linked to a theme?
- Will the finished effect be the result of a process, for example a colouring technique, a volumising technique or precision cutting, or created by the addition of specific products?
- Will your look have more impact in black and white or colour?
- What clothes and accessories are best suited to this look?
- Do you want to create natural or dramatic effects through make-up?
- Should you allow the photographer to be creative with camera angles, lighting, props and backdrops?

When you have defined your look, the plans are put into action on a story board. This will contain examples of similar looks or effects, details of styles and themes. You will need to include ideas for make-up, samples of colours and textiles. You will need to prepare a detailed plan of how each effect will be achieved, who will be involved and the running time, as well as a detailed list of all equipment and products involved. Visualising the total look and then making exhaustive preparations beforehand will save a lot of time and possibly money during the photo session.

The model

Choosing the right model is a very important factor: pretty girls are not necessarily photogenic; attractive or alluring girls may not have the right hair quality.

Professional models provide a virtually guaranteed result, but they will be very reluctant to have anything 'permanent' (such as a cut, colour or perm) done to their hair. The final effect possible will therefore be very limited. You have more scope with non-professional models, but remember, they may not be able to carry it off in front of the camera!

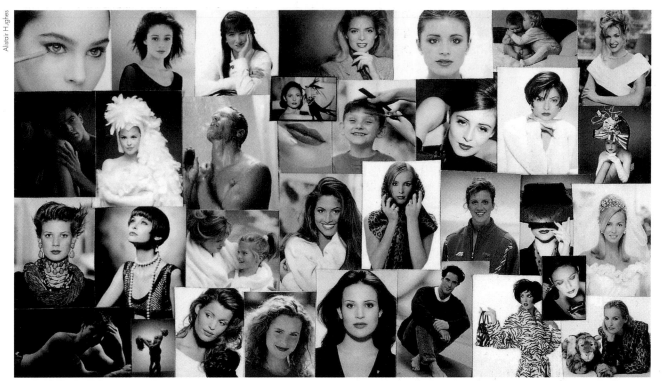

A model portfolio spread

Selecting the model

Send for portfolios of models attached to an agency. Tell them what it is for. Draw up a short list of possible models and call a casting. Take Polaroid photos and make notes. Look especially for:

- skin tone and complexion (not even the best make-up artist can hide everything)
- eye shape and colour
- quality, colour and amount of hair – bear in mind the expected purpose of the hair
- bone structure, profile, head shape and nose
- average figure (for full-length shots).

The photographer

You will need to find a photographer who specialises in hair, beauty or fashion photography. Ask to see examples of her work. Find out if she prefers to work in a studio or whether your premises can be effectively put to use (particularly useful when preparing the models). Obtain details of rates: does she charge by the hour, for half days, or for whole days only? Find out if there are additional costs for developing, duplicates or other processing. Explain what the photography is for; she will then be able to advise you on the size and format of the prints or

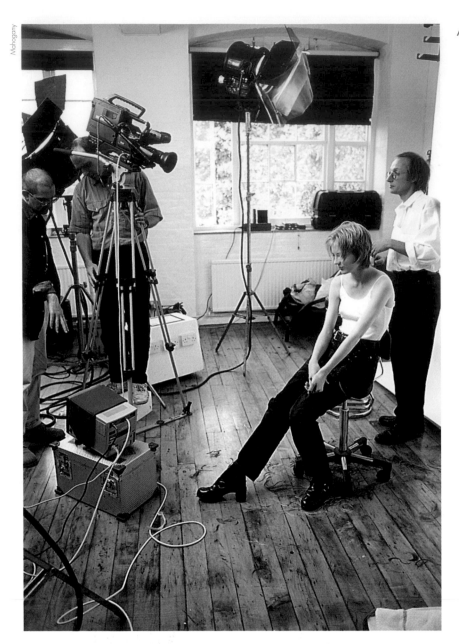

transparencies. Normally colour work for publishing will be done in 35 mm film, but other larger formats can be used for cover shots or large inclusions. Explain the look you are trying to achieve and show her the story board – she may have some useful ideas.

The make-up artist

Always use a professional make-up artist – this is vital in getting the look you require. Professional make-up artists can work quickly; they also have an eye for minute detail. Show the make-up artist examples of the effect you are trying to achieve and let her see the Polaroid shots taken at the casting – this will help her to select colours, shades and make-up effects.

Examples of different photo formats

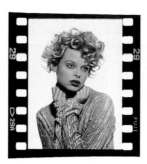

35 mm transparency

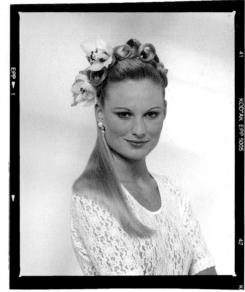

60 × 70 mm transparency

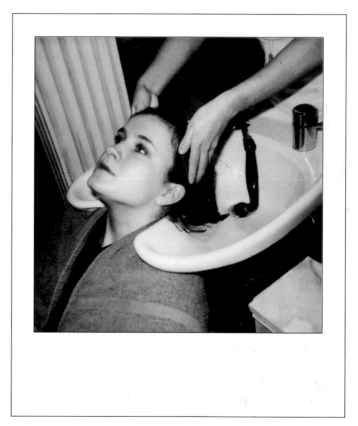

Polaroid

Clothes and accessories

Unless you are trying to achieve up-to-the-minute fashion effects, don't date your photography with the latest clothes and accessories – you should aim to create a timeless look. For head-only shots, don't clutter the camera frame with high neck lines. It is often better to show the neck and shoulders, but your main focus should be the hair.

ASSIGNMENTS

With the permission of your manager, carry out the following assignments.

1 Identify the sales and services that are most used in the salon. You can do this by making a chart listing sales and services against the days of the week.

Week 1	Mon	Tue	Wed	Thur	Fri	Sat
Cut						
Blow-dry						
Perm						
Tint						
Highlights						

Conduct this study over four weeks or more. This will show you the general trading pattern.

Pick out the day of the week on which a particular service is used least. (For example, it might be that few clients book for perms on Mondays.) Then, with the assistance of your manager, carry out a promotion based on these findings in order to increase business.

Afterwards, create another chart to evaluate the effectiveness of your promotion.

2 Arrange for a senior staff member in the salon to conduct a demonstration for the staff. Draft the plan and work through it as though the person conducting the demonstration were a visiting guest artist.

Prepare evaluation sheets for the audience to complete. How will you measure the effectiveness of the demonstration?

Using the above assignments as guidance, make notes on your work, ensuring that you document all of the aspects of promotion and demonstration. Remember to keep examples of any systems or materials that you create, for use in your portfolio.

QUESTIONS

After completing the assignments, answer these questions in your portfolio.

1 In terms of selling, what are the differences between features and benefits?

2 What methods and techniques would you use for promoting services or products?

3 What are the most effective communication techniques that should be used during hairdressing demonstrations?

4 If you were involved in the planning of a forthcoming hairdressing demonstration, how would you cater for unexpected situations?

CHAPTER 14

Health, safety and security

INTRODUCTION

This chapter looks at health, safety and security with specific relevance to:

- personal health, hygiene and appearance
- working safely in the salon
- maintaining salon security
- health and safety legislation
- writing a health and safety policy.

Legislation provided within the Health and Safety at Work Act 1974 (see page 225) requires all employees to:

> *take reasonable care for the health and safety of himself and any others who may be affected by his actions or omissions . . . and to cooperate with their employer, so that their employer can fulfil his obligation by complying with the current (UK and EC) health and safety requirements.*

It is therefore just as important to maintain personal standards of health and hygiene as to work safely in the salon.

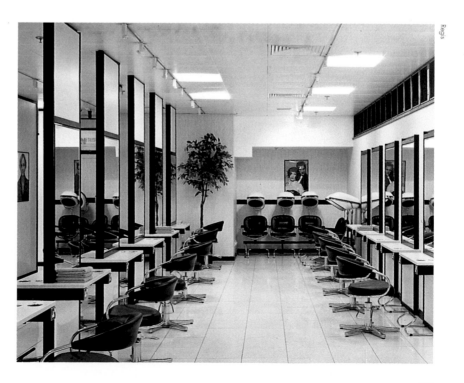

A salon

PERSONAL HEALTH AND HYGIENE

Initially, your clients will judge your personal and professional standards by the way in which you present yourself. Remember, hairdressing is an image-conscious industry. We strive to provide a high-quality service that gives clients well-cut, well-styled and well-groomed hair, so that they feel pleased and confident, and have a greater self-esteem. Would you give clients confidence if you turned up for their appointments with stained overalls, unkempt hair and dirty hands and nails?

Hands and nails

Your hands should always be perfectly clean. Dirt on your hands and under your nails will harbour bacteria. By spreading germs you could infect other people. Your hands need washing not only before work, but several times throughout the day. Where hands regularly come into contact with water or detergents, the skin may lose its moisture, become dry and crack. Cracked, broken skin allows germs to enter and infection may follow. To prevent this from happening, you should regularly moisturise your skin after washing. If your hands are often in water (for example, in shampooing or conditioning), you may find it helpful to use a *barrier cream*. Barrier creams cover the skin with an invisible barrier which greatly reduces the penetration of hairdressing cleansing and conditioning agents. (Many trainees have given up hairdressing after developing the skin condition called *dermatitis*, in which the hands become sore, cracked, itchy and red. At this stage work becomes painful and medical advice should be sought.)

Long nails not only trap dirt but can also cause discomfort to clients. In certain hairdressing procedures it is quite possible that longer nails could even scratch or damage the skin. The risk of spreading infection and disease can be prevented by keeping nails short and neat. Clean, well-manicured nails without splits or tears are hygienic and safe.

> **HEALTH AND SAFETY**
> Take all precautions to avoid dermatitis – use barrier creams and protective gloves whenever possible.

> **HEALTH AND SAFETY**
> All salons carry out a risk assessment of the substances they use. Any substances that have been identified as potentially hazardous to health will have special handling instructions. These instructions, along with any necessary personal protective equipment (PPE), must be available within the salon.

Body

Taking a daily bath is necessary to remove the build-up of sweat, dead skin cells and surface bacteria. Skin in areas such as the armpits, feet and genitals has more sweat glands than elsewhere, and the warm, moist conditions provide an ideal breeding ground for bacteria. Regular washing is therefore essential if body odour (BO) is to be prevented.

Antiperspirants will reduce under-arm sweating. These products contain astringents, which narrow the pores that emit the sweat and cool down the skin. Alternatively, *deodorants* may be used. These products will not reduce the amount of sweating but can 'mask' any odour by killing the surface bacteria with antiseptic ingredients.

Mouth

Unpleasant breath is offensive to clients. Bad breath (*halitosis*) is the result of leaving particles to decay within the spaces between the teeth. You need to brush your teeth after every meal. Bad breath can also result from digestive troubles, stomach upsets, smoking, and strong foods such as onions, garlic and some cheeses.

Personal appearance

In addition to personal cleanliness, your personal appearance is an important factor too. The effort you put into getting ready for work reflects your pride in the job. It is all right for you to have your own individual look, provided that you appreciate and accept that there are professional standards of dress and appearance that must be followed – a sort of personal code of practice.

Clothes

Clothes or overalls should be clean and well ironed. It is sensible to wear clothes made from fabrics that are suitable not only for your intended work but also for the time of year. Clothes that are restrictive or tight will not allow air to circulate around your body and will prevent you from keeping cool and fresh; they could lead to uncomfortable perspiration or possibly BO. Apart from the clothes that other people see, remember that a daily change of underwear is essential.

Shoes

Wear shoes that have low heels. They should be smart, comfortable and made of materials suitable for wearing over long periods of time. Remember that hairdressing involves a lot of standing and your feet can therefore get tired, hot, sweaty and even sore. It is worth wearing shoes that allow your feet to 'breathe', as ventilated feet remain cool and comfortable throughout the working day.

Hair

Your hair reflects the image and expected standards of the salon in which you work. It should be clean, healthy and manageable. Don't let long hair fall over your face, as this will obstruct good communication with the clients and your poor body language may give them the wrong message.

Jewellery

Only the minimum of jewellery should be worn in the salon. Rings, bracelets and dangling necklaces will get in the way of normal day-to-day duties and will make the client uncomfortable. In many hairdressing operations, such as shampooing and conditioning, jewellery can catch and pull at the client's hair as well as provide unhygienic crevices for dirt and germs to lurk in.

Posture

Bad posture will lead to fatigue or even longer-term injury. Adopting the correct posture is essential for trainee and competent hairdresser alike. An incorrect standing position will put undue strain on both muscles and ligaments, as well as giving your clients an impression of an uncaring, unprofessional attitude towards work.

Posture fatigue will occur when a part of the body is out of line with another part immediately below. Hairdressers have to be on their feet a great deal, therefore adopting a good posture is a requirement of the job. You will achieve correct posture when your head, shoulders, upper torso, abdomen, thighs and legs distribute your body's weight in a balanced, equally proportioned way, over feet that are positioned forward and slightly apart. Dropping a shoulder will shift your body's weight over one foot. This will cause curvature of the spine, applying strains on muscles and ligaments, as well as exerting pressures on the intervertebral discs in your spine. This will at least be uncomfortable and at worst dangerous, possibly starting a longer-term back problem or injury.

Your posture while sitting should be restful. Your back should be supported all the way down. This does not mean that chairs must have a continuous back or have contoured, moulded panels, but that your sitting position should provide your body with support so that the pelvis and not the base of the spine takes the body's weight.

Avoid sitting with crossed legs, as this will restrict blood circulation. It will result in numbness and a sensation of 'pins and needles'.

Infection and disease

We all carry large numbers of micro-organisms inside us, on our skin and in our hair. These organisms, such as *bacteria, fungi* and *viruses,* are too small to be seen with the naked eye. Bacteria and fungi can be seen through a microscope, but viruses are too small even for that.

Many micro-organisms are quite harmless, but some can cause disease. Those that are harmful to people are called *pathogens*. Flu, for example, is caused by a virus, thrush by a fungus and bronchitis often by bacteria. Conditions like these, which can be transmitted from one person to another, are said to be *infectious.*

The body is naturally resistant to infection; it can fight most pathogens using its inbuilt immunity system. So it is possible to be infected with pathogenic organisms without contracting the disease.

When you have a disease, the *symptoms* are the visible signs that something is wrong. They are the results of the infection and of the reactions of the body to that infection. Symptoms help you to recognise the disease.

Infectious diseases should always be treated by a doctor. Non-infectious conditions and defects can often be treated in the salon or with products available from the chemist.

GENERAL SALON HYGIENE

The salon

A warm, humid salon can offer a perfect home for disease-carrying bacteria. If they can find food in the form of dust and dirt, they may reproduce rapidly. Good ventilation, however, provides a circulating air current that will help to prevent their growth. This is why it is important to keep the salon clean, dry and well aired at all times – and this includes clothing, work areas, tools and all equipment.

A tidy salon is easier to clean. So get into the habit of clearing up your work as you go.

Floors and seating

Floors should be kept clean at all times. This means that they will need regular mopping, sweeping or vacuuming. When working areas are damp-mopped during normal working hours, make sure that adequate warning signs are provided close to the wet areas.

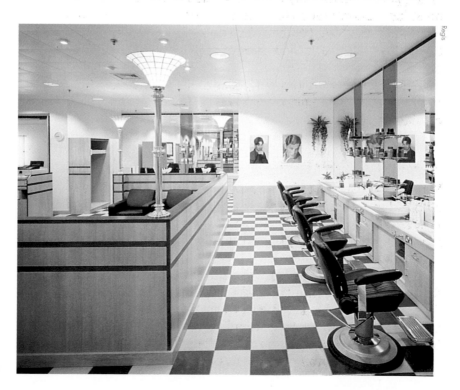

A safe, hygienic salon

(You will notice that this is a standard procedure in fast-food chains.)

The salon's seating will be made of material that is easily cleaned. It should be washed regularly with hot water and detergent. After drying, the seats can be wiped over with disinfectant or an antiseptic lotion.

Working surfaces

All surfaces within the salon, including the reception, staff and stock preparation areas, should be washed down at least once each day. Most salons now use easily maintained wipe-clean surfaces, usually some form of plastic laminate. They can be cleaned with hot water and detergent, and after the surfaces are dry they can be wiped over with a spirit-based antiseptic which will not smear. Don't use scourers or abrasives as these will scratch plastic surfaces. Scratched surfaces look dull and unattractive as well as containing minute crevices in which bacteria will develop.

Mirrors

Glass mirrors should be cleaned every morning before clients arrive. Never try to style a client's hair while she sits in front of a murky, dusty or smeary mirror. Glass surfaces should be cleaned and polished using either hot water and detergent or a spirit-based lotion that evaporates quickly without smearing.

Salon equipment

Towels and gowns

Each client must have a fresh, clean towel and gown. These should be washed in hot soapy water to remove any soiling or staining and to prevent the spread of infection by killing any bacteria. Fabric conditioners may be used to provide a luxurious softness and freshness.

Styling tools

Most pieces of salon equipment, such as combs, brushes and curlers, are made from plastics. These materials are relatively easy to keep hygienically safe, if they are used and cleaned properly.

Combs should be washed daily. When not in use they should be immersed into an antibacterial solution. When needed they can be rinsed and dried and are then ready for use.

If any styling tools are accidentally dropped on to the floor, do not use them until they have been adequately cleaned. Don't put contaminated items on to work surfaces as they could spread infection and disease.

Handle non-plastic items, such as scissors and clipper blades, with care. Clean them with surgical spirit by carefully wiping over the flat edges of the blades. Although most of these items are made of special steels, don't immerse them in sterilising fluids. Many of them contain chemicals that will corrode the precision-made surfaces of the blades.

PREVENTING INFECTION

Some salons use sterilising devices as a means of providing hygienically safe work implements. *Sterilisation* means the complete eradication of living organisms. Different devices use different sterilisation methods, which may be based on the use of heat, radiation or chemicals.

Autoclaves

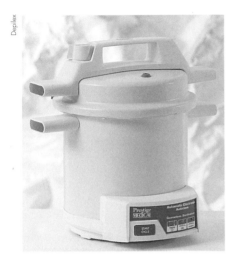

An autoclave

These provide the most effective method of sterilisation. They work on the principles of the pressure cooker. The items to be sterilised are heated with a small amount of water inside a pressurised container to a temperature of 125°C for 10 minutes. The high-temperature steam produced destroys all micro-organisms.

Ultra-violet radiation

Ultra-violet (UV) radiation provides an alternative sterilising option. The items for sterilisation are placed in wall- or worktop-mounted cabinets fitted with UV-emitting light bulbs, and exposed to the radiation for at least 15 minutes. Penetration of UV radiation is low, however, so sterilisation by this method is not guaranteed.

Chemical sterilisation

Chemical sterilisers should be handled only with suitable personal protective equipment (see page 227), as many of the solutions used are hazardous to health and should not come into contact with the skin. The most effective form of sterilisation is achieved by the total immersion of the contaminated implements into a bath of fluid. This principle is widely used in the sterilisation of babies' feeding utensils.

Disinfectants reduce the probability of infection and are widely used in general day-to-day hygienic salon maintenance. *Antiseptics* are used specifically for treating wounds. Many pre-packaged first-aid dressings are impregnated with antiseptic fluids.

WORKING SAFELY IN THE SALON

You have a duty to your employer and your colleagues to keep the working environment safe. You need to be alert, spotting potential hazards and preventing accidents, thus helping to avoid emergency situations arising. Suppose, for example, that someone had carelessly blocked a fire door with a recently delivered stock order. You could take the initiative and remove a possible hazard by moving the box to a safe and secure location. If you notice a potential hazard that you cannot easily rectify yourself, tell your supervisor immediately. Imagine, for instance, that someone accidentally tripped over a trailing lead from a hand dryer while it was plugged in, wrenching the lead from the dryer handle on to a wet floor. Under no circumstances should you enter the wet area and try to retrieve the trailing lead; but you should tell a senior member of staff at once, so that she can shut off the power at the mains supply.

Obstructions

It is dangerous to obstruct areas used as thoroughfares, such as doorways, corridors, stairs and fire exits. In an emergency, people might have to leave the salon, or part of it, in a hurry – perhaps even in the dark. It could be disastrous if someone injured themselves, or fell, in these circumstances.

So always be on the lookout for any obstruction in these areas. If you see something that could present a risk, move it away as quickly as you can.

Spillage and breakages

Take care when you have to clear up spilled chemicals or damaged equipment. First of all find out what has been spilled or dropped. Is this something that needs special care and attention when handling? Does personal protective equipment need to be worn (see page 227)?

Disposal of waste

General salon waste

Everyday items of salon waste should be placed in an enclosed waste bin fitted with a suitably resistant polyethylene bin liner. When the bin is full, the liner can be sealed using a wire tie and placed ready for refuse collection. If for any reason the bin liner punctures, put the damaged liner and waste inside a second bin liner. Wash out the inside of the bin itself with hot water and detergent.

Disposable sharps

Used razor blades and similar items should be placed into a safe screw-topped container. When the container is full it can be discarded. This type of salon waste should be kept away from general salon waste as special disposal arrangements are provided by your local authority. Contact your local council offices for more information.

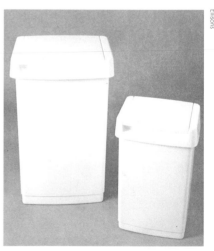

Covered waste bins

DEALING WITH ACCIDENTS

To deal with minor accidents within the salon, you need to have a basic understanding of the use of first aid. More serious injuries *must* be treated by a qualified first aider or a professional medical practitioner. The present law suggests that the ideal ratio for workplace-trained staff in low-risk occupations like hairdressing should be one trained first aider for every 50 employed (or self-employed) staff.

First-aid kit

A basic first-aid kit should consist of the following items (obviously details will depend on the number of staff employed):

- a first-aid general guidance card
- 20 assorted adhesive plasters (preferably waterproof)
- 6 medium sterile dressings
- 2 large sterile dressings (for more serious wounds)
- 6 individually wrapped triangular bandages
- 2 sterile eye pads
- a pair of scissors
- 6 safety pins
- a pair of tweezers.

In addition, the following items could prove very useful:

- antiseptic cleanser
- eye bath and eye cleansing lotion
- cottonwool
- burn ointment
- disposable bags
- disposable gloves.

Remember that any first-aid materials used from the kit must be replaced as soon as possible.

All accidents and emergency aid given within the salon must be documented in the accident book (see page 222).

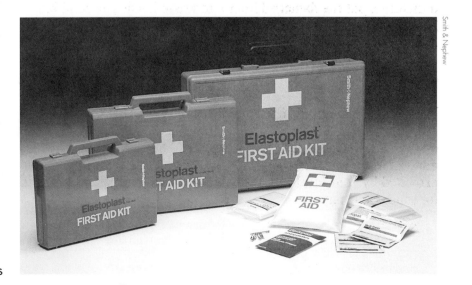

First-aid kits

General guidance on first aid

Normally a casualty should be seated or lying down when being treated by a first aider.

Problem	Action to be taken
Casualty is not breathing	**1** Place the casualty on her back. Open and clear her mouth. **2** Tilt head backwards to open airway (maintain this position throughout). Support the jaw. **3** Kneel beside casualty, while keeping head backwards. Open her mouth and pinch her nose. **4** Open your mouth and take a deep breath. Seal her mouth with yours and breathe firmly into it. Casualty's chest should rise. Remove your mouth and let her chest fall. If her chest does not rise, check her head is tilted sufficiently. Repeat at a rate of 10 times a minute until the casualty is breathing herself. **5** Place her into the recovery position.
Unconscious	Place into recovery position.
Severe bleeding	Control by direct pressure using fingers and thumb on the bleeding point. Apply a dressing. Raising the bleeding limb (unless it is broken) will reduce the flow of blood.
Suspected broken bones	Do not move the casualty unless she is in a position which exposes her to immediate danger.
Burns and scalds (due to heat)	Do not remove clothing sticking to the burns or scalds. Do not burst any blisters. If burns and scalds are small, flush them with plenty of clean, cool water before applying a sterilised dressing. If burns and scalds are large or deep, wash your hands, apply a dry sterile dressing and send the casualty to hospital.
Burns (chemicals)	Avoid contaminating yourself with the chemical. Remove any contaminated clothing which is not stuck to skin. Flush with plenty of cool water for 10–15 minutes. Apply a sterilised dressing and send to hospital.
Foreign body in eye	Wash out eye with clean cool water.*
Chemicals in eyes	Wash out the open eye continuously with clean, cool water for 10–15 minutes.*
Electric shock	Don't touch the casualty until the current is switched off. If the current cannot be switched off, stand on some dry insulating material and use a wooden or plastic implement to free the casualty from the electrical source. If breathing has stopped, start mouth-to-mouth breathing and continue until the casualty starts to breathe or until professional help arrives.
Gassing	Use suitable protective equipment. Move casualty to fresh air. If breathing has stopped, start mouth-to-mouth breathing and continue until the casualty is breathing or until professional help arrives. Send to hospital with a note of the gas involved.
Minor injuries	Casualties with minor injuries of a nature they would normally attend to themselves may wash their hands and apply a small sterilised dressing from the first-aid box.

*A person with an eye injury should be sent to hospital with the eye covered with an eye pad.

Mouth-to-mouth resuscitation procedure (see table opposite)

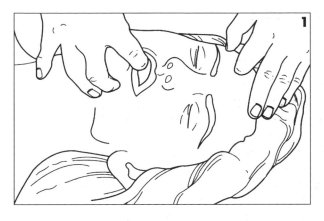

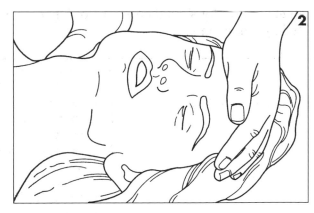

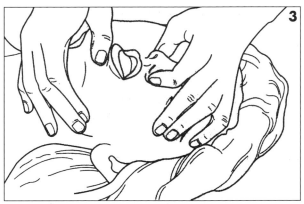

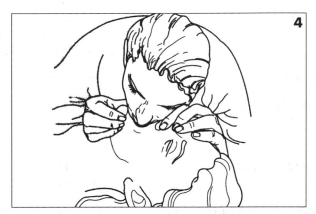

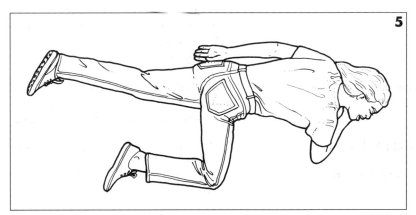

If you are fortunate, you may never need to use your first-aid skills. But you should nevertheless be prepared for the following types of incident:

- cuts
- burns
- eye injury
- sprains
- bruising
- fainting
- electric shock
- epileptic fit
- heart attack.

In a serious emergency, you could save someone's life if you knew how to give mouth-to-mouth resuscitation (see pages 220–1).

Recording accidents

All accidents must be recorded in the *accident book.* The recording system should always be kept readily available for use and inspection.

When you are recording accident details, you will need to document the following information:

- the full name and address of the casualty
- the occupation of the casualty
- the date of entry in the accident book
- the date and time of the accident
- accident details: location, circumstances, the work process involved
- injury details
- signature of the person making the entry.

FIRE

Most salon fires arise from either smoking, an electrical fault or a gas escape. *Smoking* can cause fires when lit cigarettes are dropped, discarded or left unattended to smoulder in ash trays. Faulty or badly maintained *electrical equipment,* such as hand dryers or hood dryers, may malfunction and overheat, and even ignite occasionally. *Gas appliances,* such as ovens or hobs, present a possible risk if they are left unattended. Staff cooking facilities need to be closely monitored to prevent gas being left on, whether lit or not.

Your salon will have set fire safety procedures, which must always be followed.

Raising the alarm

In the event of fire breaking out, your main priorities are to:

- *Raise the alarm* Staff and customers must be warned, and the premises must be evacuated.
- *Call the fire brigade* Do this even if you believe that someone else has already phoned. Dial 999, ask the operator for the fire service, and give the telephone number from where you are calling. Wait for the transfer to the fire service, then tell them your name and the address of the premises that are on fire.

Fire-fighting

If the fire is small, you may tackle it with an extinguisher or fire blanket.

Under the Fire Precautions Act 1971, all premises are required to have fire-fighting equipment, which must be suitably maintained in good working order.

Different types of fire require different types of fire extinguisher. For example, *never* try to use water to put out a fire caused by an electrical fault.

Fire escape

All premises must have a designated means of escape from fire. This route must be kept clear of obstructions at all times and during working hours the fire doors must remain unlocked. The escape route must be easily identifiable, with clearly visible signs. In buildings with fire certificates, emergency lighting must be installed. These lighting systems automatically illuminate the escape route in the event of a power failure and are operated by an independent battery back-up.

Fire safety training

It is essential for staff to know the following fire procedures:

- fire prevention
- raising the alarm
- evacuation during a fire
- assembly points following evacuation.

Training is given to new members of staff during their induction period. This training must be regularly updated for all staff, and fire drills must be held at regular intervals.

Fire-fighting equipment

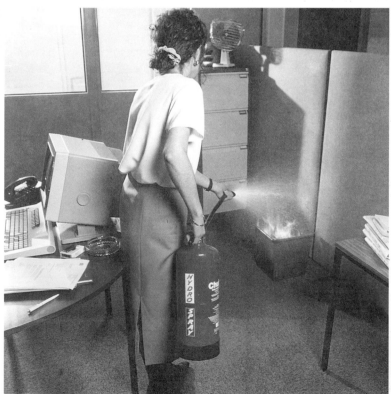

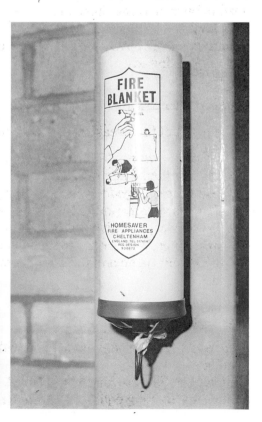

MAINTAINING SALON SECURITY

Effective salon security is essential and your employer is required by law to provide secure business premises. Moreover, insurance companies either would refuse to insure a salon where adequate precautions were not taken, or would demand premiums that were so high no salon could afford them. In order for your employer to establish and maintain the security of people and their belongings, money, equipment and premises, set procedures will have been laid down and put into action.

The potential threats to salon security come from either external or internal sources, both in and out of business hours.

External provisions

No salon can make its premises totally burglarproof, but steps may be taken to deter entry by unauthorised people and to minimise any damage they might do. As long as reasonable measures have been taken, insurance will not be withheld. Security devices should be fitted, such as:

- five-lever mortice locks ('deadlocks') to all external doors – these are locks that are rebated into (cut out of) both the door and the frame (not surface-mounted like latch locks) and which require keys to both lock and unlock them
- locking catches or bolts on all external opening windows
- security bars or grilles on potentially vulnerable points of entry
- burglar alarms that sound in the event of forced intrusion or damage.

In addition to the advised security features, particular attention should be paid to:

- never leaving money or valuables on the premises overnight
- strict control of the number and location of keys and designated key holders
- switching off all electrical or gas appliances, especially at the end of the day.

During normal hours of business, be very alert to the following risks:

- people in areas without the relevant authority
- unauthorised people asking for private or business information
- security of details relating to customers and staff.

Internal provisions

Unfortunately, outside intruders are not the only threat to the salon's security. Pilfering by staff and clients is also a possibility.

Don't let yourself think that taking the occasional product home is a 'perk' of the job. Unless it has been paid for, or you have permission, *it is theft!* Your salon may have its own policy in respect to staff purchases. Always ask.

Theft at work is defined as an act of *gross misconduct*. A thief faces instant dismissal if your employer exercises her disciplinary rights.

Your employer will have taken preventative steps to minimise the risk of theft. Procedures will be set in place to monitor till transactions, stock movements and personal items and valuables.

Money missing from the till will show up during the daily cashing up and book-keeping exercises. Shortfalls will be noticed when the number of clients attended, services and treatments provided and retail items sold do not tally with the available money and cash equivalents, the till rolls and the expected cumulative totals and the daily reports and transaction breakdowns.

Missing items of stock will be noticed during normal stock control procedures, in routine situations where stock is not available as expected, and during spot checks and searches.

The *personal possessions* of both clients and staff also need protecting from theft. Make sure that these are kept safely away from risk situations. Clients' handbags, jewellery and any other valuables should remain with them at all times. Valuable items or money belonging to staff should be securely stored during working hours, or kept with the individual, perhaps in an overall pocket.

Here is a security checklist:

- Don't leave valuables in the salon overnight.
- Don't leave money in the till.
- Leave the till drawer open overnight.
- Lock all doors, windows and cupboards.
- Secure all data/information relating to staff and clients.

HEALTH AND SAFETY LEGISLATION

This section will provide you with an outline of the main health and safety regulations that affect hairdressers and their work.

The *Health and Safety at Work Act 1974* is the legislation that covers a variety of healthy, safe working practices and associated regulations. You do not need to know the contents of this Act, but you should at least be aware of the existence of relevant regulations made under its provisions. Those that are applicable at the time of writing are as follows:

- Control of Substances Hazardous to Health (COSHH) Regulations 1988
- Personal Protective Equipment (PPE) at Work Regulations 1992
- Workplace (Health, Safety and Welfare) Regulations 1992
- Health and Safety (Display Screen Equipment) Regulations 1992
- Manual Handling Operations Regulations 1992
- Provision and Use of Work Equipment Regulations (PUWER) 1992
- Electricity at Work Regulations 1989

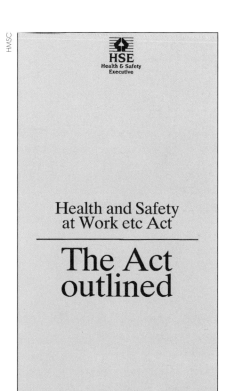

The Health and Safety at Work Act

- Reporting Injuries, Diseases and Dangerous Occurrences Regulations (RIDDOR) 1985.

Managers and employers have additional requirements that they must be able to address and/or demonstrate. But their main duty is to identify the potential hazard within the workplace, and then to eliminate the identified potential hazard to public and staff health, or minimise the risk to public and staff health by taking precautionary action.

Potential hazards are identified during *risk assessment*. This process includes:

- evaluating the processes and activities that occur at work
- recording the resulting information
- defining precautionary action to be taken.

Control of Substances Hazardous to Health (COSHH) Regulations 1988

The COSHH Regulations 1988 set out the requirements that must be observed in respect of the handling and usage of substances that are, or could potentially be, hazardous. In hairdressing terms this relates to shampoos, setting agents, perming lotions and colouring agents – all the products that we work with.

Your salon will have made a risk assessment of the products held by or used within it, and this will give you specific information on their handling and precautionary requirements.

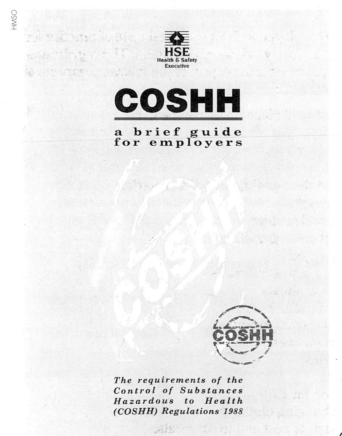

COSHH Regulations

Personal Protective Equipment (PPE) at Work Regulations 1992

The PPE Regulations 1992 require managers to make an assessment of the processes and activities carried out at work and to identify where and when special items of clothing should be worn. In hairdressing environments, the potential hazards and dangers revolve around the task of providing hairdressing services – that is, in general, the application of hairdressing treatments and associated products.

Potentially hazardous substances used by hairdressers include:

- acidic solutions of varying strengths
- caustic alkaline solutions of varying strengths
- flammable liquids, which are often in pressurised containers
- vapours and dyeing compounds.

There are also potentially hazardous items of equipment and their individual applications, such as:

- electrical appliances
- heated/heating instruments
- sharp cutting tools.

All these items require correct handling and safe usage procedures, and for several of them this includes the wearing of suitable items of protective equipment.

Workplace (Health, Safety and Welfare) Regulations 1992

These provide the employer with an approved code of practice for maintaining a safe, secure working environment. The regulations cover the legal requirements in respect of the following aspects of the working environment:

- maintenance of workplace and equipment
- ventilation
- indoor temperatures
- lighting
- cleanliness and the handling of waste materials
- room dimensions
- work stations and seating
- conditions of floor and traffic routes
- falls or falling objects
- windows, doors, gates and walls
- ability to clean windows
- organisation of traffic routes
- escalators and moving walkways
- sanitary conveniences
- washing facilities
- drinking water
- accommodation for clothing
- facilities for changing clothing
- facilities for staff to rest and to eat meals.

Health and Safety (Display Screen Equipment) Regulations 1992

Specific regulations apply to visual display units (VDUs), terminals and computer monitors. These regulations cover the safety aspects of computer operation, the accepted radiation emissions from display screens, the user's posture and seating position, along with permitted working heights.

Manual Handling Operations Regulations 1992

These regulations apply in all occupations where manual lifting occurs. They require the employer to carry out a risk assessment of the work processes and activities that involve manual lifting. The risk assessment should address detailed aspects of the following:

- any risk of injury
- the manual movement that is involved in the task
- the physical constraints the loads incur
- the (work) environmental constraints that are incurred
- the worker's individual capabilities
- steps/remedial action to take in order to minimise risk.

Provision and Use of Work Equipment Regulations (PUWER) 1992

These regulations lay down important health and safety controls on the provision and use of work equipment. They state the duties for employers, the persons in control (the users) and the self-employed. In general they affect both new and old equipment alike. In addition to this they cover the selection of suitable equipment, maintenance, manufacturer information, instruction and training. Specific regulations address the dangers that could arise from operation of the equipment and the potential risk of injury.

Electricity at Work Regulations 1989

These regulations state that electrical equipment must be adequately maintained and checked by a suitably qualified person. A written record of the equipment tests should be kept and made available for inspection.

Reporting Injuries, Diseases and Dangerous Occurrences Regulations (RIDDOR) 1985

RIDDOR requires the employer to notify the local enforcement officer, in writing, in cases where employees or trainees suffer personal injury at work. When this occurrence results in death, major injury or more than 24 hours in hospital, it must be reported by telephone first, and followed by a written report within 7 days. In all cases where personal injury occurs, an entry must be made in the salon's accident book (see page 222).

WRITING A HEALTH AND SAFETY POLICY

Writing a health and safety policy is the responsibility of any employer who has five or more employees working on the premises: this is required by law. A helpful booklet is available from your local Health and Safety Executive area office called *Writing a Safety Policy Statement: advice to employers* (ref: HSC6).

You need to draw up a general policy on health and safety, relevant to your premises. This should include:

- details of storage of chemical substances
- details of the stock cupboard or dispensary
- checks of all electrical equipment by a qualified electrician, and the details of the checks made
- names and addresses of the key-holders
- the escape routes and evacuation procedure.

It should also specify the structure of the organisation and arrangements for carrying out your policy. These should include:

- an outline of your management structure
- the name of the person responsible for health and safety in the salon
- the name of the person responsible for first aid
- the locations of the first-aid box and the accident book.

A copy of your policy should be given to each employee and the employer should ensure that they read and understand it.

ASSIGNMENTS

With the permission of your manager, carry out the following assignments.

1 Write (or review) your current health and safety policy.
2 Obtain a copy of the Health and Safety at Work Act 1974. List points relevant to your salon.
3 Carry out a study to identify potential hazards that may affect the safety of:
- members of staff
- clients and customers
- the general public.

Recommend improvements and implement agreed changes.
4 Study your security procedures for:
- staff and their belongings
- stock, both retail and product
- client's personal belongings.

Where appropriate, recommend and implement improvements to the current system.

Remember to retain any materials that you create, for use in your portfolio.

QUESTIONS

After completing the assignments, answer these questions in your portfolio.

1 What is required in health and safety checks, and why?
2 What constitutes a potential hazard? What measures should be taken to avoid potential hazards?
3 Give examples of (a) damages, (b) infestation, (c) contamination and (d) potentially unsafe features in the working environment. What remedial action should be taken to prevent each of these?
4 Give examples of possible breaches within salon security.

Portfolio guidance

WHAT IS A PORTFOLIO?

A portfolio is a 'portable statement' – a collection of your work. Whether this work has recently been undertaken or is a product of your previous experience is not important: both current and previous experiences have value. A portfolio supports your claim in seeking accreditation. It shows others (tutors, colleagues, assessors, verifiers or employers) the variety of your experience and the knowledge that you have gained.

DEVELOPING A PORTFOLIO

Preparing work in readiness for vocational qualifications will always require some written evidence. In the case of preparing for Level 3 Hairdressing, written evidence takes on a wider meaning – you won't have to write or type reams of paper, as other forms of recorded evidence are allowable. Below is an outline of a portfolio.

Description

The portfolio is a file or folder containing information which addresses specific topics in order to supplement the practical activities which have to be, or have already been, performed.

Composition

The portfolio may comprise designs, sketches, photographs, illustrations or diagrams, produced or collected by the candidate, with supporting notes.

Evidence

This will include *case studies*, which should be arranged and documented in such a way that they relate directly to the activities being performed. *Projects* and *assignments* are also required: these are similar to case studies but have clearer and more specific objectives. *Historical evidence* can be produced and should be linked to activities undertaken in the past. In many cases a personal account should be given; this is a description of the actions that have been, or that would be, undertaken. A personal account may be oral or written.

Dos and don'ts

Below are a list of simple rules to follow when you are building up your portfolio.

Do:

- be clear with explanations
- stick to the point
- keep to the assessment requirements
- explain procedures step by step
- use your creativity, including designs or sketches
- make use of photography or illustrations
- ask others to validate or give testimony
- cross-refer where applicable
- ask your tutor if you need help
- use a variety of types of evidence.

Dont:

- pad out or lengthen topics
- leave your work incomplete
- lose your work – it's valuable!

Remember, pieces of information, small in themselves, can turn into valuable evidence.

EXAMPLES OF SUPPLEMENTARY EVIDENCE

Portfolios record evidence. This doesn't necessarily mean that you have to write, type or otherwise record all the information in your portfolio: there are many forms of evidence that you can simply collect to support your projects and assignments. Below is a list of documents and systems that you may wish to use:

- completed forms and questionnaires
- checklists
- agendas and minutes
- reports
- diaries and appointment books
- action plans
- computer printouts
- job appraisals
- job specifications
- letters
- costings and budgets
- charts and graphs
- rotas
- record cards.

These forms of evidence are collectively referred to as 'historical evidence'. You may also make use of authenticated 'products of experience': wigs and hairpieces, even videos of past demonstrations or competitions.

Accreditation of prior learning (APL)

Many candidates who wish to obtain the NVQ Level 3 in Hairdressing are, or have been, hairdressers working in salons without any formal qualifications. Many of these candidates may have extensive vocational skills and experience, already equivalent to current Level 3 standards. It would be a waste of time and money to enrol these individuals on to a preset training programme, when all they require is an assessment system that will identify existing competences and highlight any areas where 'top-up training' is required.

Candidates choosing to take this route towards qualification should get in touch with their nearest Level 3 training centre so that a personal action plan can be devised to meet their needs.

Useful addresses

The organisations listed below should prove valuable sources of information and help to the professional hairdresser. Address any enquiries to 'The Secretary'.

Arbitration, Conciliation and Advisory Service (ACAS)
Clifton House, 83–117 Euston Road, London NW1 2RB
(Tel. 0171-396 5100)

Black Beauty and Hair
Hawker Publications,
13 Park House, 140 Battersea Park Road, London SW11 4NB
(Tel. 0171-720 2108)

Caribbean and Afro Society of Hairdressers (CASH)
42 North Cross Road, East Dulwich, London SE22 8PY
(Tel. 0181-299 2859)

City and Guilds
1 Giltspur Street, London EC1A 9DD
(Tel. 0171-294 2468)

Cosmetic, Toiletry and Perfumery Association (CTPA)
Josaron House, 5–7 John Princes Street, London W1M 9HD
(Tel. 0171-491 8891)

The Fellowship for British Hairdressing
Waterloo House, High Street, Tisbury, Wiltshire SP3 6HD
(Tel. 01747 870310)

Freelance Hair and Beauty Federation
6 Warleigh Road, Brighton, East Sussex BN1 4NT
(Tel. 01273 604556)

Guild of Hairdressers (GUILD)
Meadowhall Hairdressing and Beauty Supplies, Unit 8, Vulcan Road, M1 Distribution Centre, Meadowhall, Sheffield S9 1EW
(Tel. 0114-242 2454)

Hair and Beauty/Hair Now/Your Salon
109/110 Bolsover Street, London W1P 7HF
(Tel. 0171-436 9766)

Hair Magazine
IPC Magazines Ltd, King's Reach Tower, Stamford Street, London SE1 9LS
(Tel. 0171-261 5000)

Hairdressers Journal International
Quadrant House, The Quadrant, Sutton, Surrey SM2 5AS
(Tel. 0181-652 3500)

Hairdressing Council (HC)
12 David House, 45 High Street, South Norwood, London SE25 6HJ
(Tel. 0181-771 6205)

Hairdressing Employers Association (HEA)
10 Coldbath Square, London EC1R 5HL
(Tel. 0171-833 0633)

Hairdressing Manufacturers' and Wholesalers' Association (HMWA)
Bedford Chambers, The Piazza, Covent Garden, London WC2E 8HA
(Tel. 0171-836 4008)

Hairdressing Training Board (HTB)
2nd Floor, Fraser House,
Nether Hall Road,
Doncaster, DN1 2PH
(Tel. 01302 380000)

Institute of Trichologists
20–22 Queensberry Place,
London SW7 2DZ
(Tel. 0171-491 7253)

National Hairdressers Federation (NHF)
11 Goldington Road, Bedford MK40 3JY
(Tel. 01234 360332)

Union of Shop, Distributive and Allied Workers (USDAW)
188 Wilmslow Road, Fallowfield,
Manchester M14 6LJ
(Tel. 0161-224 2804)

World Federation of Hairdressing and Beauty Schools
PO Box 367, Coulsdon, Surrey CR5 2TP
(Tel. 01737 551355)

asymmetrical Unevenly balanced; without an equal distribution of hair on either side.

balance The effect of hair shape on the features of the face and head; even proportions.

baseline An initial cutting line from which later cutting lines are established.

basing cream A form of skin protection used when perming or straightening hair.

bleaching Removing colour from hair.

body language Communicating by means of body actions and/or posture rather than words.

cashier The person responsible for transactions at the point of payment.

club cutting Cutting a hair section straight across, producing blunt ends.

collodion A protective covering used in skin testing.

colour depth Lightness or darkness of hair colour.

colour-filling Applying a preliminary colouring of red to hair so that new colour will adhere.

communication The exchange of information and the establishment of understanding between two people, as for example between the stylist and the client.

compensation Providing money or services to offset a deficiency and make amends.

complainant Someone who expresses dissatisfaction or a grievance.

computerised Operated automatically using electronic apparatus.

concave Sloping inwards.

concept An idea, impression or thought.

confidential Private information; not for general use.

consultation A process of communication in which the client expresses her wishes and the hairdresser gives advice.

contraindication A reason why a proposed course of action or treatment should not be pursued.

convex Sloping outwards.

creative Individual ability to make a form, shape or style which ideally enhances.

databank A manual or computerised store of data or records.

decolouring Removing synthetic colour from hair.

demonstration A display and explanation of a physical instruction.

depilatory Designed to remove hair.

designer Creator of images.

diagnose Determine the condition of the hair and scalp.

disclaim To renounce or reject legal responsibility.

endorsement A signature in confirmation of some statement, affirming that it is true.

eumelanin A natural hair pigment.

formative assessment A tool for the regular monitoring and review of students' progress, and a means of regular dialogue between trainee and tutor. Formative assessments indicate when a trainee is ready for a summative assessment.

franchise Authorisation to sell company goods or services in a specified area.

graduation A sloping variation from long hair to short, or from short to long, produced by cutting the hair ends at a particular angle.

hair extension Real or synthetic fibre added to existing hair.

hair strand A section of hair; a mesh, tress or piece.

historical evidence Evidence resulting from activities that have been undertaken in the past.

host company A company that authorises others to operate – similar to a franchising company, but with more direct involvement in daily procedures.

image Likeness; what is seen or portrayed; overall appearance.

incentives Rewards for effort.

incompatible Causing a chemical reaction on mixing, as between a chemical being added to the hair and another chemical already on the hair.

induction The familiarisation process that staff undergo when they first join an organisation. (This may include health and safety requirements.)

lightening Removing colour from hair.

line The line of a style is determined by the directions in which the hair is positioned.

lye The common name for sodium hydroxide.

manually By hand.

merchandise Goods for sale.

movement Variation of the line of a style, such as waves.

negotiation The process of reaching agreement by discussion.

non-verbal communication Means of communication other than words – gestures, facial expressions, stance, and so on.

occipital Bone forming the back of the head.
originality New; created for the first time; the ability to be original or inventive.
ornamentation Flowers, ribbons, jewellery and the like, worn to enhance the hairstyle.

parietal Bones forming the upper sides of the head.
perimeter The outside line of the hair.
personality The mannerisms, habits, ways and characteristics of a person – individual identity.
pheomelanin A natural hair pigment.
physiognomy The general appearance of the head and face.
porosity The ability to hold moisture.
portfolio A file or folder containing evidence that supports practical activities that have been carried out previously.
postiche A dressed hairpiece.
pre-pigmenting Applying a preliminary colouring of red to hair so that new colour will adhere.
promotion Advertising by way of a publicity campaign.

quality assurance The process by which a desired outcome is guaranteed by means of monitoring and verification.
quality management The establishment and implementation of systems and procedures relating to each function and task, and to personnel, to ensure consistency.
quality standard Required criteria for a function or part of a function.

recolouring Adding further colouring to hair.
relaxing Reducing the curl or wave in hair.
resources Means of supplying needs (people, stock or facilities).

senses The means by which we see, hear, touch, smell and taste.
serrations The saw-like edges of some scissors.
stabiliser A chemical added to hydrogen peroxide to maintain its strength, for example phosphoric or sulphuric acid.
straightening Reducing the curl or wave in hair.
summative assessment A means of final evaluation of a trainee's competence against the standards indicated by the stated performance criteria. This is usually carried out when it is felt that a trainee has reached the desired level of competence for a particular element.
symmetrical Balanced by means of an even and equal distribution of hair on either side.
synthetic Artificially made; not natural.
systems Procedures; ways in which things are carried out.
systems manual A book, file or folder displaying the complete system for each aspect of procedure.

tapered Thinner towards the hair points.

tariff A displayed list of fixed charges.

temporal Bones forming the lower sides of the head.

tension The stress or stretch experienced by hair.

texture The feel or appearance of the hair – rough, smooth, coarse or fine.

textured Shaped to take account of the fineness or coarseness of hair, giving lift and fullness.

toning Adding colour to bleached hair.

traction Stress or pull applied to hair.

traction baldness An area of baldness resulting from the stress or pull applied to hair.

training techniques Approaches to training – demonstration, observation, private study, and so on.

transaction The execution of a specific task, together with payment for this task.

void To make invalid.

whorls Hair growth patterns.

accessories   16, 139, 209
accident book   171, 222, 228
acid perms   75–6
acne   32
action plan   151
activators (bleaching)   111
added hair   129–39
advertising   204
Advisory Conciliation and Arbitration
   Service (ACAS)   166
African-Caribbean techniques   143–50
   consultation   143
   hair type   6
   relaxing hair   146–50
   styling using heated equipment   144–5
age, client's   23
albinism   35
alkaline perms   75–6
allegorical   22
allocating work   162–3
alopecia   32
appointment book   151, 162
appraisal   156–60
artificial colouring   105–6
Asian hair   6
assessment   192–8
   assignments   196
   collecting evidence   196–7
   continual   192
   feedback   197–8
   oral   197
   recording   198
   written   197
asymmetric shimmer   96–7
asymmetrical cutting   63–4
autoclaves   217
automatic tills   175
avant-garde   22

bacterial infectious diseases   29–30
baldness   32
banking   174
basing   147
bigoudies   74
bleaching   110–15
   chemistry   111
   choice of bleach   112–13
   methods   114–15
   problems and solutions   109, 112
   variations   113
blending fibres   134–5
blepharitis   33
block colouring   100–1
block highlights   90–1
body language   154–5
body shape   14

canities   35
cape wiglet   129
card payments   176–7
cleaning hairpieces   131–2
cashpoint   174–7
Caucasian   6
charge cards   177
chemical sterilisation   217
cheques   176
chignon   129
chopsticks   87
client
   age   23
   care   68–9
   complaints   25
   consultation   18
   expectations   21
   information   20
   late arrival   152
   legislation   225
   lifestyle   14, 21
   treatment records   184
clippers   66

closed questions   197
clothes and accessories   16, 209
club cutting   64
code of practice   165, 227
cold perming   75
colour   15, 104–6
   chart   105
   depth   104
   flashes   94–5
   mixing   104–6
   selection   104–6
   shades   105
   spectrum   104
   synthetic extensions   134–5
   test   27, 110
   tone   104
colouring   89–118
   bleaching   110–12
   decolouring   118
   methods   113–15
   principles   104–6
   problems and solutions   109, 116–17
   recolouring   115–16
   toning   116
colourants   106–8
common cold   30
communication   153–5
complaints   25
competence   192
components of standards   193–5
computerised cash desk   175
concave cutting   63
conditions, hair and scalp   32–3
confidentiality   19
conjunctivitis   33
consultation   18–36
contingency planning   161–2
continual assessment   19
Control of Substances Hazardous to Health
   (COSHH) Regulations   70, 172, 226
   accidents   171, 219, 222
   employee's responsibilities   211
   health and safety policy   229
   preventing infection   217
convex cutting   63
cornrowing   128
Cosmetic, Toiletry and Perfumery
   Association (CTPA)   172
credit cards   177
crimpers   87
cross-infection   69
curl check or test   27
curlers   79
Customs and Excise   173
cutting   37–70
   accuracy   67
   asymmetrical   62–3
   baselines   62–3, 68
   checks   67–8
   health and safety   69–70
   symmetrical   62
   texturising   66–7
   tools   63–6

dandruff   33
day book   179
day sheet   178–9
decolouring   118
defects, hair and scalp   34–5
demonstrations   183, 202–4
depth of colour   104
dermatitis   32, 212
directional perm   82
disciplinary action   164–6
diseases, hair and scalp   29–31
disposal of waste   218
dressing hair   119–42
duties of employers, health and safety
   225–9

essential knowledge   195
element of competence   193
eczema   32
exothermic   74
elasticity test   28, 110
equal opportunities   164
extensions, hair   132–9
   synthetic fibre   133–7
   processed natural hair   137–9
eye contact   154
eumelanin   104, 110
European hair   6

face and head shapes   11
facial expression   10
facial framing   102–3
feedback   197–8
finance   173–81
   cashpoint   174
   methods of payment   176
   records   177
   systems   173
   VAT   178–9
fire   222–3
   fighting   222
   safety training   223
Fire Precautions Act   222
first aid   219–22
flea   31
float   176
folliculitis   30
formal meetings   155
formal training activities   196
formers   86
fragilitas crinium   34
franchise   173
frosting   113
fungal infectious diseases   30–1
furunculosis   29

gestures   154–5
gift vouchers   176
graduated bob   38–41
graduation
   forward   58–62
   short   50–3
   short contemporary   42–5
grievance procedure   166

hair
   accessories   139
   added, postiche   129–32
   colourants   104
   diseases, conditions and defects   29–35
   extensions   132–9
   growth patterns   5, 24, 62
   movement   4, 66, 81
   pigmentation   104
   quality and quantity   4–6, 10, 24, 62
   tests   26–8, 110
   type   6, 143
Hairdressing Manufacturers' and
   Wholesalers' Association (HMWA)
   172, 233
hands   13, 212
haute coiffure   22
health and safety   211–29
   employee responsibilities   171, 215–22
   employer responsibilities   171–2, 211,
      224–9
   legislation   211, 225–9
   personal health   212–15
   policy   229
   preventing infection   217
   salon hygiene   215–17
   security   224–5
Health and Safety at Work Act   225
herpes simplex   30
herpes zoster   30
high knot   120–1

highlighting 113
historical styling 22
hot perming 74
human resources 168
hydrogen peroxide 111–12
hypersensitivity 26

image 1–2, 9–17
impetigo 29
incompatibility test 28, 110
infections 29–31, 214
influenza 30
informal meetings 155
information 155
Inland Revenue 173

jewellery 214
job description 158

knots 120–3

layered colour 92–3
learning
    directed 182
    student-centred 183
    flexible 184
legislation, health and safety 211, 225–9
lice 31
lifestyle 14, 21
lightening 110
line management 174
line of style 3
longer-lasting colourants 107
low knot 122–3
lowlighting 113
lye 146

mailshot (direct marketing) 201
maintaining records 151
make-up 13, 17, 208
manual tills 175
marteaux 129
measuring effectiveness 157
meetings 155
melanin 104
memorandum 153–4
Mongoloid 6
monilethrix 35
monitoring 186, 201
Monofibre™ extensions 133–6
motivation 190
mouth-to-mouth resuscitation 220–1
movement 4, 66, 81

natural hair extensions 137–9
neck and shoulders 13
neutralising colour 106, 116
non-verbal communication 154–5
normalising perms 80–1

open questions 197
oral communication 153
oral assessment 197
ordering stock 170–1
organisational policy 151, 165
ornamentation 139–40
overbleaching 112
overbooking 152

parasites, hair and scalp 31
pediculosis capitis 31
performance
    appraisal 156–60
    criteria 194
    evidence 196–7
    records 196
perimeter 3, 63
permanent colourants 107
perming 71–88

equipment 78, 84, 86–8
    lotion choice 82
    normalising 80
    problems and solutions 81, 83
    systems 74–8
    techniques 78–88
    winding 79, 85–8
peroxide test 27
perruquier 74
Personal Protective Equipment (PPE) at
    Work Regulations 227
personality 14, 23
petty cash book 174, 180
pheomelanin 104, 110
photography 205–9
physical features 22
physical resources 169–73
pincurls 129
pityriasis capitis 33
plaiting 126–8
planning
    contingency 161–2
    staff cover 161
    training 185–6
pleat 124–5
polymerisation 107
porosity 143
    test 28, 110
portfolio 197, 230–1
post-damping 76, 79
postiche 129–32
posture 154, 214
pre-damping 76, 79
pre-pigmenting 115
presentations 183
preventing infection 217
product application 8
product coding 170
productivity 180–1
promotion 199–210
psoriasis 33
pulex irritans 31

Qualifications and National Curriculum
    Authority (QCA) 192
quality and quantity of hair 4–6, 10, 24, 62
quasi-permanent colourants 107

razor cut 65
razors 64
reception 19
recolouring 115
recorded evidence 197
recording accidents 222
relaxing hair 146–50
resources 168–80
    financial 173–80
    human 168
    physical 169–73
    time 168
resuscitation, mouth-to-mouth 220–1
ringed hair 35
rods 79
role-play 184
root perming 78

scabies 31
scissors 63–4
sebaceous cyst 35
seborrhoea 33
security 172, 174, 224–5
self-appraisal 159, 190
self-development 190
self-discipline 191
self-organisation 191
semi-permanent colourants 107
seminars 183
senses 1

shades 105
sharps, disposal of 218
shelf-life (stock) 169
skin test 26, 110
spillage 218
spiral curls 78–81
square layers 54–7
staff
    absences 152
    appraisals 156–60
    attitudes 163
    cover 161
    records 159, 161
    relationships 155–6
    supporting 163
    training 182–9
standards of competence 192
stock control 169–73
straightening hair 144–5
strand test 27, 110
style artistry 1–8
styling hair 119–42
summative assessment 196
supervisor, role of 160–4
supplementary evidence 231
surface slices 98–9
swathes 129
switches 129
sycosis 29
symmetrical cutting 62–3
synthetic fibre extensions 133–6

team working 151–67
temporary colourants 106
test curl 27
test cutting 27
texture 4, 24
texturising 66–7
theft and damage 172, 224–5
thinning scissors 63
tills 151, 175
time resources 168
tinea capitis 30
tinea pedis 31
tipping colour 113
tones 104–5
toning 116–17
torsades 129
traction baldness 32
training 182–91
    assessment 184–5
    delivering 187–8
    methods 183–4
    planning 185–6
    schedule 188
    sources 182
transient short layers 46–9
traveller's cheques 176
trichologist 32–3
trichorrhexis nodosa 34
twisting 120–1

U-stick rods 88
under-plaiting 128
underpinning knowledge 192

value-added tax (VAT) 178–9
verrucae 30
viral infectious diseases 30
volume 66

warts 30
waste disposal 218
weave winding 84
weaving 128–9
winding techniques 85–8
Workplace (Health, Safety and Welfare)
    Regulations 227